PRESS HERE!

CHAKRAS
~FOR BEGINNERS~

PRESS HERE!

CHAKRAS
~FOR BEGINNERS~

A SIMPLE GUIDE TO BALANCING YOUR ENERGY CENTERS

VICTOR ARCHULETA

FAIR WINDS

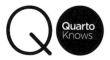

Inspiring | Educating | Creating | Entertaining

Brimming with creative inspiration, how-to projects, and useful information to enrich your everyday life, Quarto Knows is a favorite destination for those pursuing their interests and passions. Visit our site and dig deeper with our books into your area of interest: Quarto Creates, Quarto Cooks, Quarto Homes, Quarto Lives, Quarto Drives, Quarto Explores, Quarto Gifts, or Quarto Kids.

© 2020 Quarto Publishing Group USA Inc.

First Published in 2020 by Fair Winds Press, an imprint of The Quarto Group.

100 Cummings Center, Suite 265-D, Beverly, MA 01915, USA. T (978) 282-9590 F (978) 283-2742

Fair Winds Press titles are also available at discount for retail, wholesale, promotional, and bulk purchase. For details, contact the Special Sales Manager by email at specialsales@quarto.com or by mail at The Quarto Group, Attn: Special Sales Manager, 100 Cummings Center, Suite 265-D, Beverly, MA 01915, USA.

23 22 21 20 24 1 2 3 4 5

ISBN: 978-1-59233-941-9

Digital edition published in 2020

QUAR.328316

Conceived, edited, and designed by Quarto Publishing plc. 6 Blundell Street, London N7 9BH

Editor: Claire Waite Brown
Senior art editor: Emma Clayton
Designer: Joanna Bettles
Illustrator: Kuo Kang Chen
Publisher: Samantha Warrington

Printed in Singapore.

The information in this book is for educational purposes only. It is not intended to replace the advice of a physician or medical practitioner. Please see your health-care provider before beginning any new health program.

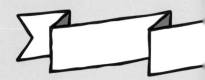

Welcome   6

The Benefits of Chakra Balancing   8

About This Book   10

Chapter 1

BASIC PRINCIPLES OF CHAKRA BALANCING   12

What are Chakra Energy Centers?   14

Where are the Seven Primary Chakras?   16

Intention and Willingness   18

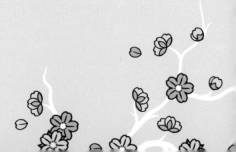

CONTENTS

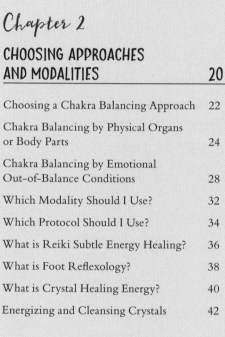

Chapter 2

CHOOSING APPROACHES AND MODALITIES 20

Choosing a Chakra Balancing Approach 22

Chakra Balancing by Physical Organs or Body Parts 24

Chakra Balancing by Emotional Out-of-Balance Conditions 28

Which Modality Should I Use? 32

Which Protocol Should I Use? 34

What is Reiki Subtle Energy Healing? 36

What is Foot Reflexology? 38

What is Crystal Healing Energy? 40

Energizing and Cleansing Crystals 42

Chapter 3

CHAKRA BALANCING PROTOCOLS 44

The Root Chakra 46

The Sacral Chakra 56

The Solar Plexus Chakra 66

The Heart Chakra 76

The Throat Chakra 86

The Third-eye Chakra 96

The Crown Chakra 106

Chapter 4

RESOURCES 116

Chakra Reference Table 118

Ailments Directory 120

Index 126

Acknowledgments 128

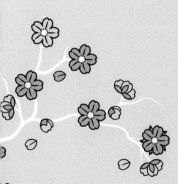

WELCOME

HAVING AN AWARENESS OF THE EXISTENCE OF THE SEVEN MAIN CHAKRA ENERGY CENTERS ENABLES US TO CHECK IN AND EVALUATE THE STATE OF EACH. ONCE YOU ARE AWARE OF WHICH CHAKRAS ARE OUT OF BALANCE, YOU CAN DETERMINE AN APPROACH FOR REALIGNING THEM. THIS BOOK PROVIDES AN UNDERSTANDING OF HOW TO USE REIKI, FOOT REFLEXOLOGY, AND CRYSTAL ENERGY TECHNIQUES TO BALANCE YOUR CHAKRAS.

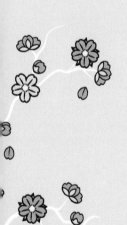

THE BUSY AND SOMETIMES FRENETIC PACE OF 21ST-CENTURY LIVING CAN MAKE IT CHALLENGING TO MAINTAIN BALANCE AND CLARITY IN OUR EVERYDAY LIVES. WE TRY TO DO IT ALL, BUT IT CAN OFTEN BE AN UPHILL BATTLE. WHILE WE CAN BE SUPER ORGANIZED AND DISCIPLINED TO ACCOMPLISH EVERYTHING WE WANT TO ACHIEVE, WE SOMETIMES FALL SHORT. BY MAKING A COMMITMENT TO OUR WELLNESS, WE CAN ACTUALLY ACHIEVE MORE OF OUR GOALS WITH GRACE AND EASE IN A BALANCED AND MORE FOCUSED WAY. READERS CAN UTILIZE THE CHAKRA BALANCING PROTOCOLS PRESENTED IN THIS BOOK AS PART OF AN OVERALL WELLNESS PLAN.

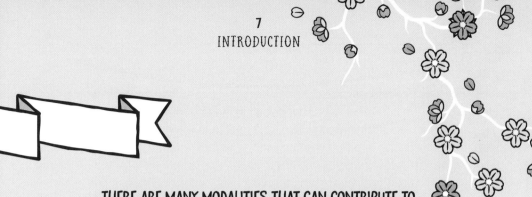

THERE ARE MANY MODALITIES THAT CAN CONTRIBUTE TO YOUR OVERALL WELLNESS, INCLUDING YOGA, MEDITATION, PRAYER, AND EXERCISE. ALL OF THESE HAVE THE EFFECT OF DECREASING STRESS BY INCREASING RELAXATION. THE GOAL IS TO BRING ABOUT A STILLNESS IN WHICH THE BODY IS IN A DEEPLY RELAXED, SELF-HEALING STATE. ADDING CHAKRA BALANCING TECHNIQUES TO YOUR TOOLKIT MAY HELP YOU ACHIEVE THIS STILLNESS AND BEGIN THE PROCESS OF UNWINDING, UNTWISTING, AND RELEASING ENERGETIC OR PHYSICAL "KINKS" IN THE BODY'S NATURAL FLOW.

Victor E. Archuleta

VICTOR ARCHULETA

DISCLAIMER

This book is not intended to diagnose illness or disease, nor is it meant to prescribe treatments for curing illness or disease. Wherever the words "heal" or "healing" appear, it is intended that the protocols themselves do not "heal," but rather facilitate the body's own ability to heal itself. While many of these protocols may be useful, it is important to note that they are generally not supported by scientific research or evidence-based studies. Any physical or mental health challenges you may be experiencing should be addressed by a qualified physician and/or psychotherapist. The reiki information presented in this book is not intended as a substitute for training by a reiki master, and the methodologies and protocols presented should only be utilized as a gift to the readers themselves and to their loved ones.

THE BENEFITS OF CHAKRA BALANCING

By understanding the myriad ways in which your chakra energy centers are affected, you can focus your awareness and utilize a number of modalities to align, balance, and strengthen them for increased vitality and overall well-being. By applying techniques from various wellness modalities, you will attempt to achieve deep relaxation and tension relief. This will facilitate the body's ability to self-correct and improve many of the symptoms that occur when chakras are out of balance.

Along with a robust toolkit that includes reiki subtle energy therapy, reflexology, and crystal healing, you will utilize your imagination to incorporate mindfulness, philosophy, and color to maintain balanced chakras. Being empowered with a number of choices, you can make the necessary adjustments that may alleviate some of the most common ailments you may experience.

Balanced chakras will bring you closer to your goal of relieving tension, restoring vitality, and improving flow to various body systems, thus facilitating your body's natural ability to heal itself.

Some of the many benefits of utilizing the chakra balancing protocols detailed in this book may include:

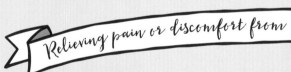

Relieving pain or discomfort from

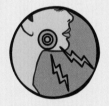

LOWER BACK PAIN   JAW PAIN

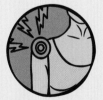

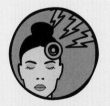

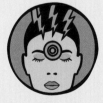

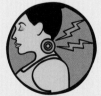

SHOULDER PAIN   HEADACHES   MIGRAINES   NECK PAIN

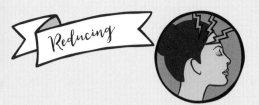
Reducing

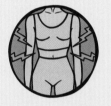
ANXIETY

DEPRESSION

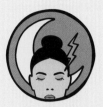
FATIGUE/
RESTLESSNESS/
INSOMNIA

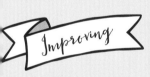
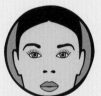
BODY STRESS/STRAIN/
TENSION

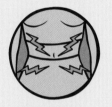
DIGESTIVE
IRREGULARITY

Improving

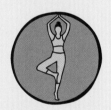
CLARITY AND
FOCUS

FLEXIBILITY AND
RANGE OF MOTION

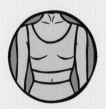
OVERALL
WELL-BEING

Achieving

DEEP RELAXATION

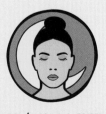
DEEP/RESTFUL SLEEP

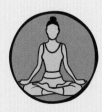
CALM MIND/BODY

ABOUT THIS BOOK

This book will guide the reader through a simple step-by-step process to determine which chakras may be out of balance, which modality is most appropriate for the issue(s) being addressed, and the techniques for performing the rebalancing of the chakra. By using a multi-modality approach to chakra balancing, the reader is empowered to undertake the steps needed to rebalance one or more of the seven energy centers.

①
Basic Principles of Chakra Balancing

PAGES 12-19

Here you will learn what chakras are, where they are located, and how to prepare yourself for balancing them.

②
Choosing Approaches and Modalities

PAGES 20-43

In this chapter you will find out how unbalanced chakras manifest and the approaches you can use to rebalance them.

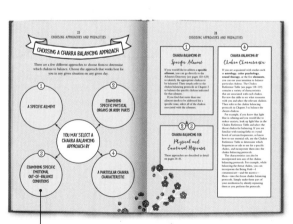

PHYSICAL AND EMOTIONAL CONDITIONS

HERE YOU WILL LEARN HOW TO SPOT THE SIGNS THAT A CHAKRA IS OUT OF BALANCE.

3

Chakra Balancing Protocols

PAGES 44-115

This chapter guides you through the protocols that can be used to balance each chakra, and details how you know when a particular chakra is unbalanced.

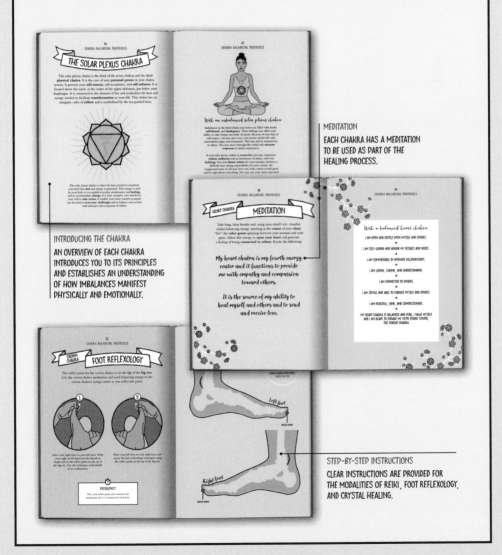

MEDITATION
EACH CHAKRA HAS A MEDITATION TO BE USED AS PART OF THE HEALING PROCESS.

INTRODUCING THE CHAKRA
AN OVERVIEW OF EACH CHAKRA INTRODUCES YOU TO ITS PRINCIPLES AND ESTABLISHES AN UNDERSTANDING OF HOW IMBALANCES MANIFEST PHYSICALLY AND EMOTIONALLY.

STEP-BY-STEP INSTRUCTIONS
CLEAR INSTRUCTIONS ARE PROVIDED FOR THE MODALITIES OF REIKI, FOOT REFLEXOLOGY, AND CRYSTAL HEALING.

1

BASIC PRINCIPLES OF CHAKRA BALANCING

WHAT ARE CHAKRA ENERGY CENTERS?

Each of the seven chakras corresponds to physical neurologic ganglia
or plexuses along the spine that influence nearby endocrine glands
and organs. Generally, the understanding is that there are energetic
pathways that spiral from the top of the head, down the spine to the
sacrum, and back up to the head. The back-and-forth spirals form
points of intersection at specific locations in the head and along the
spine. Chakra energy centers reside at these intersecting points.

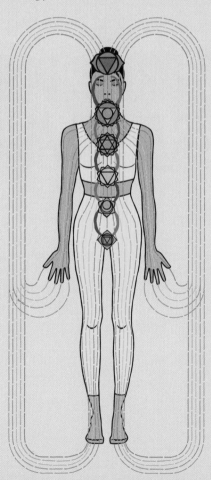

BASIC PRINCIPLES OF CHAKRA BALANCING

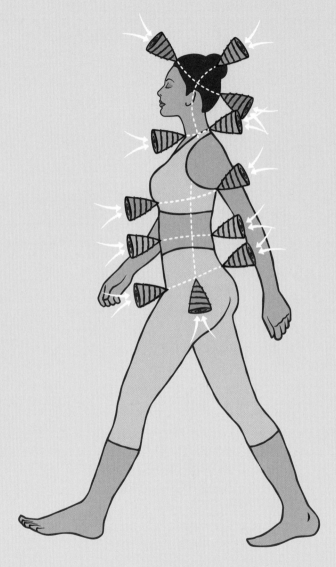

Energy centers occur as spinning vortices and patterns that have been studied
and documented in ancient Ayurvedic and Chinese medicine. In Western
wellness circles, these energy centers are commonly known as chakras.

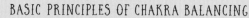

WHERE ARE THE SEVEN PRIMARY CHAKRAS?

THE FIRST CHAKRA IS THE ROOT CHAKRA, LOCATED AT THE BASE OF THE SPINE.

★

THE SECOND CHAKRA IS THE SACRAL CHAKRA, LOCATED BELOW THE NAVEL AND AROUND THE SACRUM.

★

THE THIRD CHAKRA IS THE SOLAR PLEXUS CHAKRA, LOCATED AROUND THE SOFT BELLY, ABOVE THE NAVEL AND BELOW THE RIB CAGE.

★

THE FOURTH CHAKRA IS THE HEART CHAKRA, LOCATED AT THE CENTER OF THE CHEST AROUND THE HEART.

★

THE FIFTH CHAKRA IS THE THROAT CHAKRA, LOCATED AT THE BASE OF THE THROAT ABOVE THE COLLARBONES.

★

THE SIXTH CHAKRA IS THE THIRD-EYE CHAKRA, LOCATED AT THE CENTER OF THE FOREHEAD JUST ABOVE AND BETWEEN THE EYEBROWS.

★

THE SEVENTH CHAKRA IS THE CROWN CHAKRA, LOCATED AT THE TOP OF THE HEAD.

BASIC PRINCIPLES OF CHAKRA BALANCING

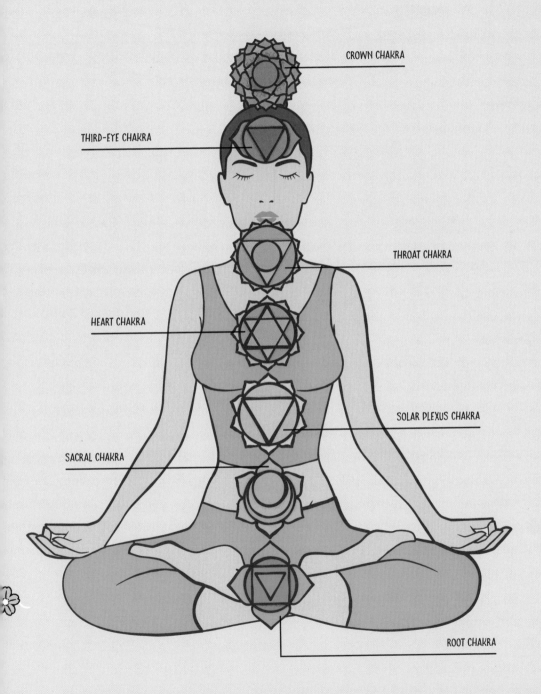

CROWN CHAKRA

THIRD-EYE CHAKRA

THROAT CHAKRA

HEART CHAKRA

SOLAR PLEXUS CHAKRA

SACRAL CHAKRA

ROOT CHAKRA

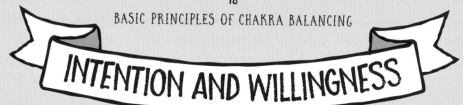

INTENTION AND WILLINGNESS

Chakra balancing work depends on focused intention and willingness. Your intention is critical to invoking the flow of energy. This, combined with your willingness to accept the energy flow, allows the process to proceed. Through your commitment to your well-being, the flow of subtle energy is invoked. As in any meditation practice, we are able to access subtle energies in the quiet silence of stillness.

Setting your Intention

There is no right or wrong way to do the work. With the appropriate intention and willingness, subtle energy will go to work with little to no effort on anyone's part. It is important not to be attached to an outcome or a result. Trust and allow.

Centering/Grounding

By centering and grounding yourself, and meditating on your intentions, you bring awareness to the vital consciousness that drives your chakra energy centers and brings balance and harmony to this energy system.

Meditation

Chakra balancing work does not happen in a vacuum. Meditation that includes visualization and reciting affirmations sets the stage for the work to be done. It communicates your conscious and specific intentions for your own well-being.

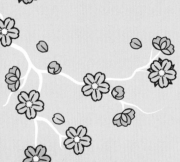

I AM...

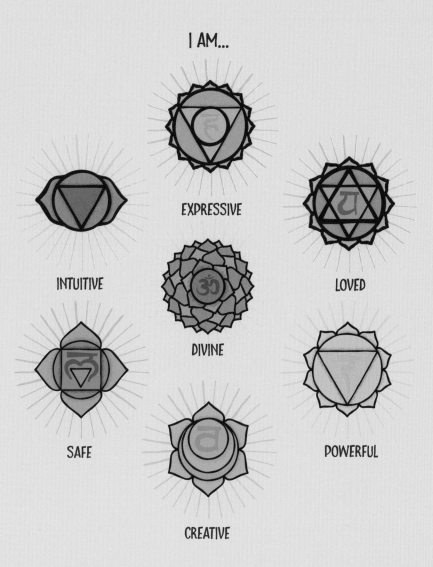

EXPRESSIVE

INTUITIVE

LOVED

DIVINE

SAFE

POWERFUL

CREATIVE

By using the meditations, recitations, and affirmations included in each of the chakra balancing protocols in Chapter 3, you create an energetic field that will facilitate your chakra balancing effort.

2
CHOOSING APPROACHES AND MODALITIES

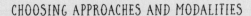

CHOOSING A CHAKRA BALANCING APPROACH

There are a few different approaches to choose from to determine which chakras to balance. Choose the approach that works best for you in any given situation on any given day.

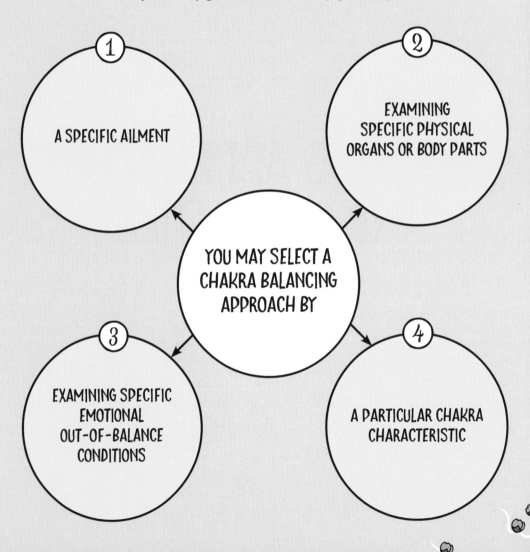

CHAKRA BALANCING BY
Specific Ailment

If you would like to address a **specific ailment**, you can go directly to the Ailments Directory (see pages 120–125) to identify the appropriate chakras to be balanced. Then simply refer to the chakra balancing protocols in Chapter 3 to balance the specific chakras indicated for that ailment.

If you find that more than one ailment needs to be addressed for a specific issue, select all of the chakras associated with the ailments.

CHAKRA BALANCING FOR
Physical and Emotional Responses

These approaches are described in detail on pages 24–31.

CHAKRA BALANCING BY
Chakra Characteristic

If you are acquainted with studies such as **astrology**, **color psychology**, **sound therapy**, or the five **elements**, you can use your intuition to balance particular chakras. The Chakra Reference Table (see pages 118–119) contains a variety of characteristics that are associated with each chakra. Review the table to see what resonates with you and select the relevant chakras. Then refer to the chakra balancing protocols in Chapter 3 to balance the chosen chakras.

For example, if you know that light blue is calming and you would like to reduce anxiety, look up light blue in the Chakra Reference Table and select the throat chakra for balancing. If you are familiar with tuning forks or crystal bowls of certain frequencies, or know how to use essential oils, use the Chakra Reference Table to determine which frequencies or oils to use for a specific chakra, and incorporate them into the chakra balancing protocols.

The characteristics can also be incorporated into any of the chakra balancing protocols. For example, while balancing the throat chakra, you can incorporate the Being Verb—I communicate—and the mantra—Ham—into the throat chakra balancing protocols. Simply make them part of your meditation by silently repeating them as you perform the protocols.

CHAKRA BALANCING BY PHYSICAL ORGANS OR BODY PARTS

If you are well acquainted with your own body you may already know where you are physically out of balance. If so, you only need to know what the corresponding chakra is for a particular physical organ or body part.

Use the summary on the following pages that specifies the major organs and body parts associated with each chakra to help identify which chakras to address. Because endocrine glands are powerful regulators of major organs and body systems, their associations with each chakra are identified separately, along with their regulatory functions.

Once you have identified which chakras to rebalance, refer to the chakra balancing protocols in Chapter 3 to balance the chakras for the specific physical organ, gland, or body part you want to address.

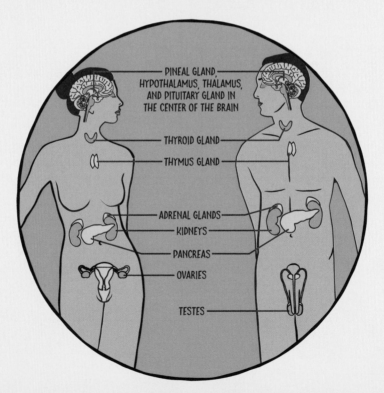

PINEAL GLAND,
HYPOTHALAMUS, THALAMUS,
AND PITUITARY GLAND IN
THE CENTER OF THE BRAIN

THYROID GLAND

THYMUS GLAND

ADRENAL GLANDS
KIDNEYS

PANCREAS

OVARIES

TESTES

Root Chakra

ENDOCRINE GLAND	ORGANS / BODY PARTS
Adrenal glands Regulate metabolism and the immune system	Colon, anus, rectum, testes/prostate (m), legs, feet

Sacral Chakra

ENDOCRINE GLAND	ORGANS / BODY PARTS
Adrenal glands Reproductive glands (testes in men; ovaries in women) Regulate sexual development and secrete sex hormones	Colon, anus, rectum, testes/ovaries, legs, feet

Solar Plexus Chakra

ENDOCRINE GLAND	ORGANS / BODY PARTS
Pancreas Regulates metabolism	Abdomen, lower back, stomach, pancreas, spleen, liver, gallbladder, intestines

Heart Chakra

ENDOCRINE GLAND	ORGANS / BODY PARTS
Thymus gland Regulates the immune system	Thoracic cavity, heart, upper back, rib cage, chest, circulatory system, lungs

Throat Chakra

ENDOCRINE GLAND	ORGANS / BODY PARTS
Thyroid gland Regulates body temperature and metabolism	Mouth, jaw, ears, throat, vocal cords, neck, trachea, thyroid, shoulders, arms, hands

Third-eye Chakra

ENDOCRINE GLANDS	ORGANS / BODY PARTS
Pituitary gland Produces hormones and governs the function of the previous five glands Thalamus gland Involved in sensory perception and regulation of motor functions Hypothalamus gland Produces hormones and works with the pituitary and thalamus glands to regulate a number of body systems and functions	Eyes, nose, sinuses, medulla

Crown Chakra

ENDOCRINE GLAND	ORGANS / BODY PARTS
Pineal gland Regulates biological cycles, including sleep (Note: the pineal gland is sometimes linked to the third-eye chakra as well as the crown chakra.)	Brain, cerebral cortex, cranium

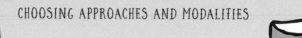

CHAKRA BALANCING BY EMOTIONAL OUT-OF-BALANCE CONDITIONS

If you would like to take an approach that addresses emotional rather than physical imbalances, then you will need to know how your feelings relate to a particular chakra.

Use the summary below to compare your own feelings to those emotional conditions related to overactive and underactive chakras. Once you have determined which chakras to address, refer to the chakra balancing protocols in Chapter 3 to balance the chakras you have identified.

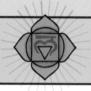

Root Chakra Emotional Conditions	
OVERACTIVE	**UNDERACTIVE**
Conditions of an overactive root chakra may include feelings of distrust or **paranoia**. Fear-based emotions contribute to **anxiety**. You may be obsessed with trying to protect yourself.	Conditions of an underactive root chakra may include feelings of extreme **vulnerability** and withdrawal. Lethargy and disconnection contribute to **loneliness** and hopelessness. You may feel depressed and stuck in a "funk" with no way out.

Sacral Chakra Emotional Conditions

OVERACTIVE	UNDERACTIVE
Conditions of an overactive sacral chakra may include **unhealthy feelings** around your **sexuality**. You may be obsessed with **material wealth** and **blocked creatively**.	Conditions of an underactive sacral chakra may include feeling **repressed** and **ashamed** around your **sexuality**. You are unable to create abundance in your life and unable to maintain a healthy, intimate relationship.

Solar Plexus Chakra Emotional Conditions

OVERACTIVE	UNDERACTIVE
Conditions of an overactive solar plexus chakra may include the need to **control** and intimidate **others**. You may be manipulative and even **condescending** because of your overly inflated sense of self.	Conditions of an underactive solar plexus chakra may include feelings of **inadequacy** because you lack the confidence to take action. You may constantly seek the **approval of others** and easily give up your power to those around you.

Heart Chakra
Emotional Conditions

OVERACTIVE	UNDERACTIVE
Conditions of an overactive heart chakra may include being **quick to fall in love** with no clear foundation for doing so. You may be **codependent** and tend to take on the problems of the world.	Conditions of an underactive heart chakra may include feelings of depression, **loneliness**, and a **lack of empathy**. You may respond by being passive-aggressive, **selfish**, and **unable** to **love yourself**.

Throat Chakra
Emotional Conditions

OVERACTIVE	UNDERACTIVE
Conditions of an overactive throat chakra may include **speaking without thinking** through what you are trying to communicate. You may shout when speaking because you **don't feel heard** or understood.	Conditions of an underactive throat chakra may include a speech impediment or the **inability to speak in public**. You may appear shy and unconfident, speaking softly or **mumbling** when sharing your thoughts.

Third-eye Chakra Emotional Conditions

OVERACTIVE	UNDERACTIVE
Conditions of an overactive third-eye chakra may include **delusional thinking** and an overreliance on intellect rather than intuition when evaluating your world. You may feel **superior** to others and become **arrogant** and authoritative.	Conditions of an underactive third-eye chakra may include being blind to what is plain and clear to others. Not trusting or believing in your intuitive sense, you may **not** be able to **visualize your path** or make plans to create your future.

Crown Chakra Emotional Conditions

OVERACTIVE	UNDERACTIVE
Conditions of an overactive crown chakra may include being **obsessed** with finding your **spiritual path** without really grasping the fundamentals of who you are. You may harm your body by believing that you are serving a higher spiritual calling.	Conditions of an underactive crown chakra may include feelings of isolation because of your **inability to connect** with others in a deep and **spiritual way**. You may be dogmatic in your certainty that atheism is the only truth.

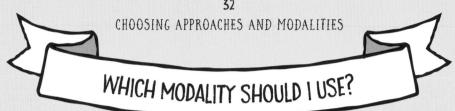

WHICH MODALITY SHOULD I USE?

Because of the energetic nature of the chakra system, there are actually a variety of modalities that can be used to balance each chakra. To realign out-of-balance conditions for a particular chakra, it can sometimes be more effective to address these conditions from multiple angles. Using more than one approach for a particular condition may provide a greater opportunity to achieve rebalancing.

The intention of this book is to provide an easy-to-use, step-by-step process, so it focuses on the **first three** of these **modalities**: reiki, foot reflexology, and crystal healing energy. The protocols of these three modalities are simple, **effective**, **easy to understand**, and do not require a lot of knowledge to apply.

The modality protocols do have slightly different approaches in their application. Reflexology utilizes direct physical contact, applying pressure to specific reflex points to achieve the desired result, while reiki uses light, gentle touch, and even hovering, to balance a chakra energy center. And although crystal healing energy has physical contact with the body at the chakra energy center, this modality largely relies upon visualizing the energy of a particular crystal working to balance the chakra.

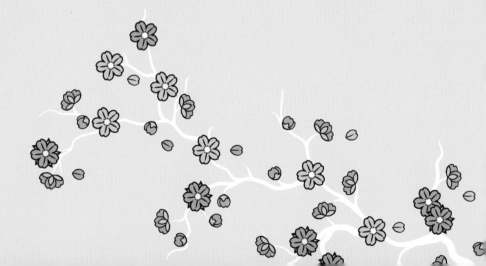

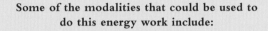

Some of the modalities that could be used to do this energy work include:

REIKI

Subtle energy healing using the hands
to channel the Universal Life Energy

REFLEXOLOGY

Utilizes hand techniques to apply pressure
to specific body map reflex points

CRYSTAL HEALING ENERGY

Utilizes energetic frequencies from minerals

ESSENTIAL OILS

Utilizes aromatherapy from plant-based oils

YOGA AND PRANAYAMA

Utilizes body movements with specific breathing techniques

MEDITATION

Utilizes quiet stillness while observing your thoughts

MANTRAS

Utilizes short repeated phrases in meditation

YANTRAS

Utilizes gazing at specific images along with mantras

MUDRAS

Utilizes specific hand and finger positions along
with mantras and yantras

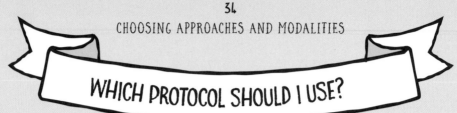

WHICH PROTOCOL SHOULD I USE?

You can use a single protocol or a mix of all three protocols, depending on what you want to achieve. Look at this chart to help you choose which to use.

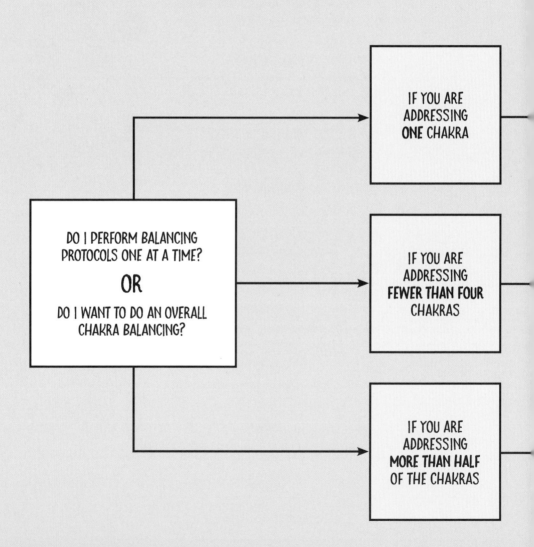

IF YOU ARE ADDRESSING **ONE** CHAKRA

DO I PERFORM BALANCING PROTOCOLS ONE AT A TIME?

OR

DO I WANT TO DO AN OVERALL CHAKRA BALANCING?

IF YOU ARE ADDRESSING **FEWER THAN FOUR** CHAKRAS

IF YOU ARE ADDRESSING **MORE THAN HALF** OF THE CHAKRAS

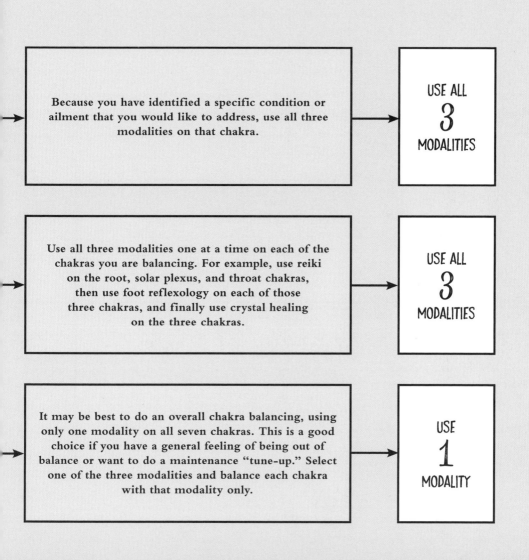

Because you have identified a specific condition or ailment that you would like to address, use all three modalities on that chakra.

USE ALL
3
MODALITIES

Use all three modalities one at a time on each of the chakras you are balancing. For example, use reiki on the root, solar plexus, and throat chakras, then use foot reflexology on each of those three chakras, and finally use crystal healing on the three chakras.

USE ALL
3
MODALITIES

It may be best to do an overall chakra balancing, using only one modality on all seven chakras. This is a good choice if you have a general feeling of being out of balance or want to do a maintenance "tune-up." Select one of the three modalities and balance each chakra with that modality only.

USE
1
MODALITY

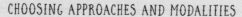

WHAT IS REIKI SUBTLE ENERGY HEALING?

Usui Shiki Ryoho is a specific form of reiki practice that allows the student to have contact with the energy of reiki simply by laying on of hands in self-treatment and the treatment of others. This system of practice is described in the philosophy and understanding of the Four Aspects and Nine Elements, defined in the teachings of Mikao Usui, Chujiro Hayashi, Hawayo Takata, and Phyllis Furumoto.

Reiki is a Japanese concept translated as "Universal Life Energy." The phrase was coined by Mikao Usui to describe the energy that he had contacted through years of self-preparation and dedication.

The following description of reiki is taken from Hawayo Takata's journal when she was a beginner student of Chujiro Hayashi, circa 1935.

66 *The power is unfathomable, immeasurable, and being a universal life force, it is incomprehensible to man.* 99

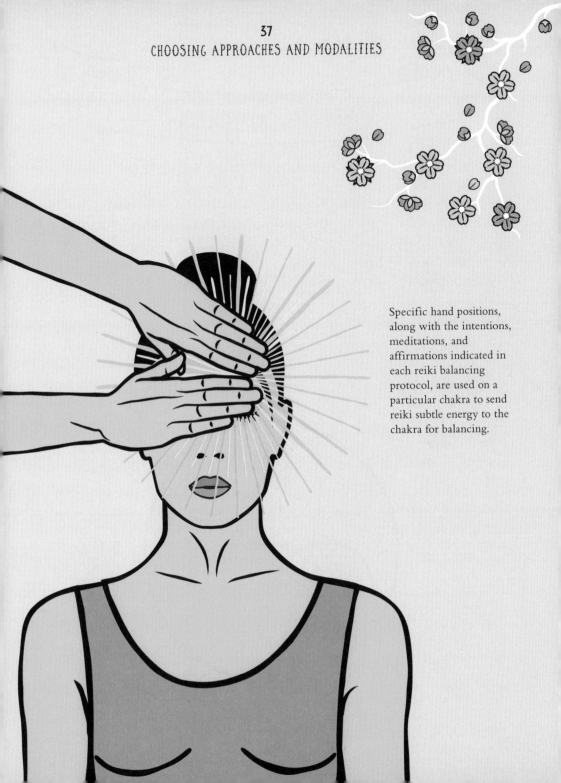

Specific hand positions, along with the intentions, meditations, and affirmations indicated in each reiki balancing protocol, are used on a particular chakra to send reiki subtle energy to the chakra for balancing.

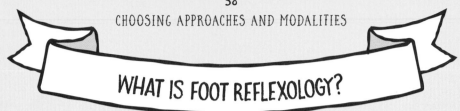

WHAT IS FOOT REFLEXOLOGY?

Foot reflexology is performed using gentle, relaxing finger and thumb movements on specific reflex points on the feet. Theory suggests that a map corresponding to various parts of the human body exists on the top, bottom, and sides of each foot. Some of these reflex points also correspond to each of the seven chakras. Wide ranges of health benefits have been reported from using foot reflexology.

Finger and Thumb Rolls

Various finger and thumb movements are used to reflex a specific chakra reflex point on the foot. In this book we use a thumb or finger roll.

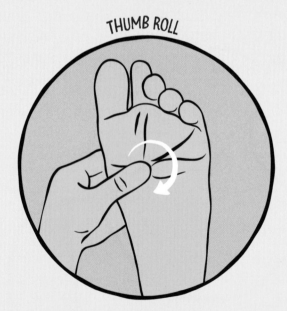

THUMB ROLL

Use your thumb to gently press the reflex point and make a circular/rolling motion to apply light pressure. Think of the reflex point being the size of a bottle cap.

> " *If you're feeling out of kilter, don't know why or what about, let your feet reveal the answer, find the sore spot, work it out.* "
>
> Eunice D. Ingham, founder of reflexology

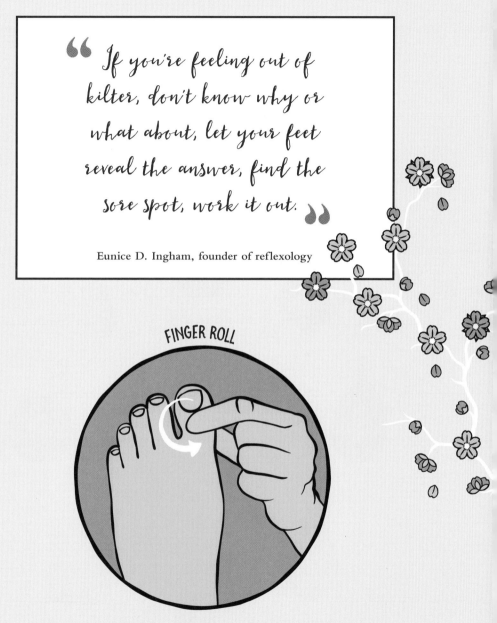

FINGER ROLL

Use your index finger to gently press the reflex point and make a circular/rolling motion to apply light pressure. Think of the reflex point as being the size of a bottle cap.

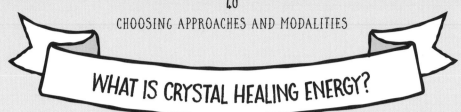

WHAT IS CRYSTAL HEALING ENERGY?

Crystals have long been used for a variety of wellness purposes.
They can be placed on your body, worn as parts of jewelry,
or carried in pouches to receive the benefits of their particular
energetic frequencies.

Choosing Crystals

You may use the crystals specified in the
protocols for each chakra in Chapter 3, or
you may simply choose crystals that are the
same color as the chakra you would like to
balance. The effectiveness is greatly
influenced by your intention.

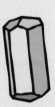

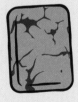

Crystals can be placed on the body or
held in the hand and, along with the
specific intentions, meditations, and
affirmations indicated in Chapter 3, be
used to balance each of the seven chakras.

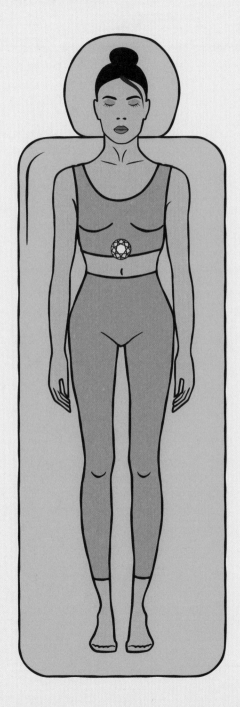

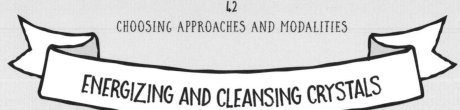

ENERGIZING AND CLEANSING CRYSTALS

Through repeated use crystals can pick up denser energies, so they benefit from regular cleansing and reenergizing. There are a number of ways to do this. Cleansing and energizing should be done when you first acquire your crystals, and can then take place on a regular basis, with the frequency depending on how often you use them.

CAUTION

Many crystals will fade in direct sunlight, so sun baths should be restricted to clear or white crystals. Moonlight, on the other hand, is not harmful to any crystals.

Do not use the water bath technique for halite, selenite, and desert rose because they are very soft and will melt in the water. Also, bloodstone, hematite, lodestone, and malachite will rust because of their iron content. If you are at all unsure about a particular crystal, do not cleanse or energize with water.

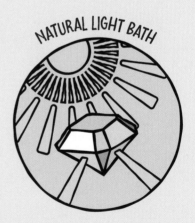

NATURAL LIGHT BATH

Use the natural energy of the sun—see Caution—or the full moon (day before, day of, and day after) to cleanse and charge your crystals. Place the crystals on a clean surface and allow the sunlight or moonlight to bathe them. Leave for one to two hours during the day or overnight for a moon bath.

SMUDGING

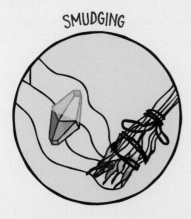

Burn incense of sage, sweetgrass, sandalwood,
or palo santo. Place the crystals on a clean
surface and smudge for a few minutes,
allowing the smoke to waft above them.
You can use a feather to help direct the
smoke toward the crystals.

CRYSTAL GEODE CAVE/CLUSTER

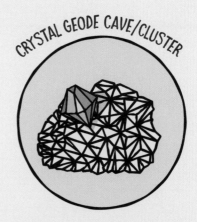

Amethyst, selenite, and clear quartz can be
used to cleanse and energize your crystals.
You can place crystals inside a geode of
amethyst or quartz, or on top of larger
crystals of selenite or quartz clusters.
Allow to purify for a few hours.

SALT

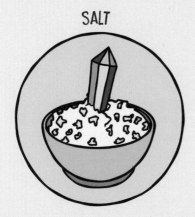

Use dry sea salt without water. Fill a small
bowl with Himalayan sea salt and place the
crystal on the surface of the salt, or bury it just
beneath the surface. Leave to cleanse and
charge overnight. The following day, gently
rinse with cool filtered water and dry with
a soft cloth.

WATER BATH

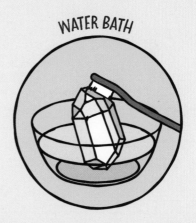

Dip crystals—see Caution—in a bowl of cool
filtered water without sea salt (sea salt in water
can cause corrosion of certain crystals and is
not recommended for cleansing), then, using a
soft toothbrush, gently brush the surfaces and
nooks and crannies. Remove from the water
bath and dry gently with a soft cloth.

3

CHAKRA BALANCING PROTOCOLS

THE ROOT CHAKRA

The root chakra is the first of the seven chakras and the first **physical chakra**. It is the foundation of the chakra system. It governs your feelings of safety, **survival**, and **security**. It is located near the perineum, at the base of the spine between the genitals and the anus. It is physically closest to the **earth** and links you to the **physical world**. This chakra has an energetic color of **red** and is symbolized by the four-petaled lotus.

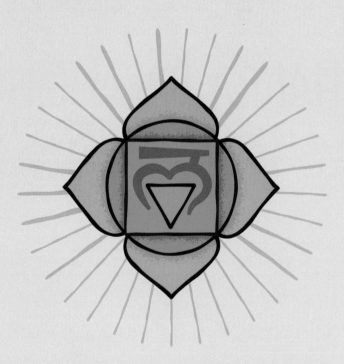

The root chakra is the first chakra to develop in the womb and in the first year of life. It drives your will to survive in the material world. This energy center powers your fight-or-flight impulse. When properly developed, you will feel **safe**, **nurtured**, and **connected** to yourself, your family, and community.

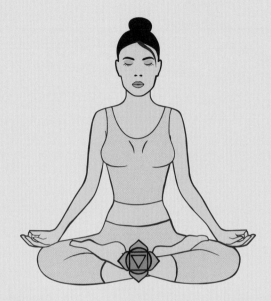

With an unbalanced root chakra

Imbalances in the first chakra may leave you feeling light-headed, **spacey**, and even **dizzy**. These imbalances may be situational or related to historical trauma, such as child neglect, abuse, and even a difficult birth. Chronic ailments from the hips down may result. Because you are not grounded in the physical world, you may be left with feelings of danger and **uncertainty**.

If the root chakra is **overactive** you may experience a sense of **anxiety** or **paranoia**. You may worry unnecessarily and be plagued by catastrophic thinking, such as fear of losing your job, home, or relationship. The world around you will often seem chaotic and unmanageable. Because of feelings of **scarcity** you may compensate by becoming greedy, competitive, and judgmental, and see life as a zero-sum game of winners and losers.

If the root chakra is **underactive** you may feel **powerless** and **disconnected** from the world, losing your ability to trust those around you. You may feel victimized in an "us versus them" view of the world. You may even be afraid of the dark or afraid to be alone for no apparent reason. You might have feelings of hopelessness and **depression**, and even have suicidal thoughts, seeing no way out of situations you feel were imposed upon you.

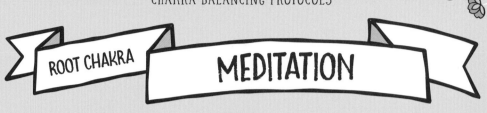

ROOT CHAKRA — MEDITATION

Take long, deep breaths and, using your mind's eye, visualize chakra balancing energy spinning at the **base** of your **abdomen** and "see" the **color red** spinning between your genitals and your anus. Allow this energy to ground and center you. Recite the following:

My root chakra is my first energy center and it functions to ground me energetically to the earth.

This is my connection to the physical world.

My trust and security rest here.

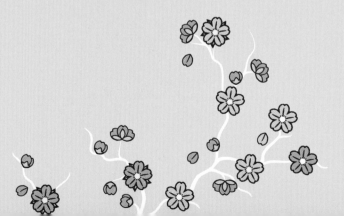

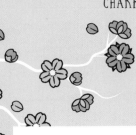

With a balanced root chakra

ALL OF MY BASIC NEEDS ARE BEING MET.

★

I AM SAFE AND SECURE.

★

I AM STABLE AND CONNECTED TO MY BODY
AND TO THE EARTH.

★

I AM CALM AND AT PEACE.

★

I AM CONNECTED AND SAFE IN THE WORLD.

★

I AM TRUSTING AND ALLOWING LIFE TO UNFOLD.

★

MY ROOT CHAKRA IS BALANCED AND VITAL. I AM COMFORTABLE
AND READY TO ENGAGE MY SECOND ENERGY CENTER,
THE SACRAL CHAKRA.

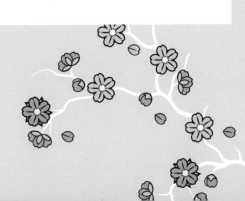

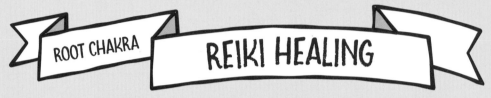

ROOT CHAKRA
REIKI HEALING

Use the root chakra meditation and visualize the Reiki Universal Life Energy flowing as you hold these hand positions.

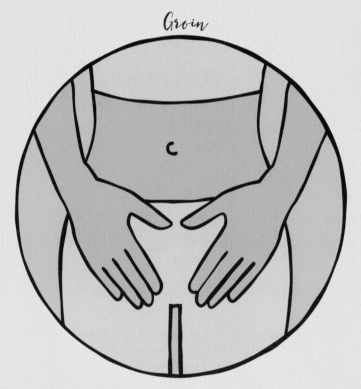

Close your eyes and cup your hands. With your palms facing you and your fingertips facing downward and inward, place your hands on your lower abdomen. Gently press the base of your palms on your hips.

FREQUENCY

Hold each hand position and continue the meditation for 2–3 minutes.

See also

WHAT IS REIKI SUBTLE
ENERGY HEALING?
PAGES 36–37

ROOT CHAKRA MEDITATION
PAGES 48–49

Coccyx

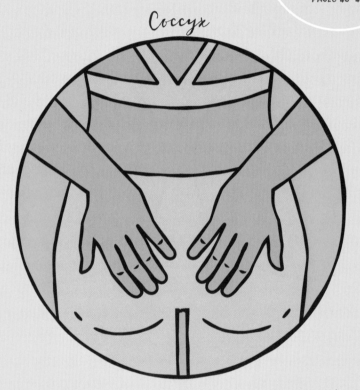

Close your eyes and cup your hands. With your palms facing you and your
fingertips pointing downward and inward, place your hands behind you, on
the top and center of your buttocks. Gently press your little fingers
on your sacrum.

ROOT CHAKRA FOOT REFLEXOLOGY

The reflex point for the root chakra is on the **inside edge** of the
foot on the **heel**. Use the root chakra meditation and send balancing
energy to the chakra's energy center as you reflex the point.

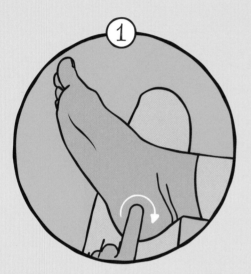

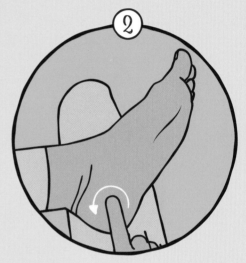

Place your right foot on your left knee.
With either hand use the thumb or finger
roll on the reflex point on the inside edge
of the heel. Use the techniques individually
or in combination.

Place your left foot on your right knee and
repeat the foot reflexology technique on the
reflex point on the inside edge of the heel.

FREQUENCY

Flex each reflex point and continue
the meditation for 2–3 minutes for
each foot.

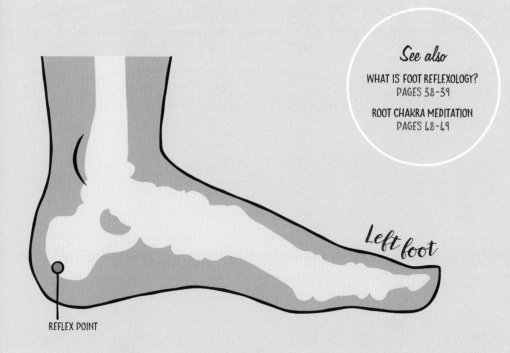

See also

WHAT IS FOOT REFLEXOLOGY?
PAGES 38-39

ROOT CHAKRA MEDITATION
PAGES 48-49

Left foot

REFLEX POINT

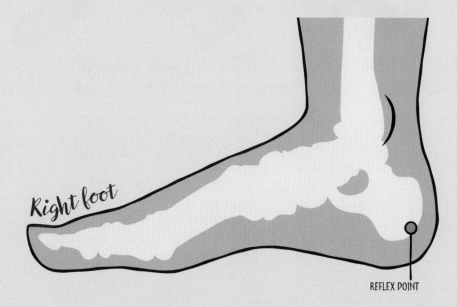

Right foot

REFLEX POINT

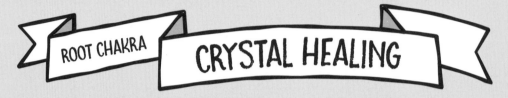

ROOT CHAKRA

CRYSTAL HEALING

Place your chosen crystal on the root chakra location on the pubic bone—you can also simply hold the crystal in your left hand. Use the root chakra meditation to send healing energy from the crystal to the root chakra energy center.

Selection process

Choose a crystal corresponding to the root chakra.

GARNET

RUBY

BLACK TOURMALINE

See also

WHAT IS CRYSTAL
HEALING ENERGY?
PAGES 40-41

ROOT CHAKRA MEDITATION
PAGES 48-49

TO BALANCE THE ROOT CHAKRA,
YOU CAN PLACE THE CRYSTAL ON
THE PUBIC BONE.

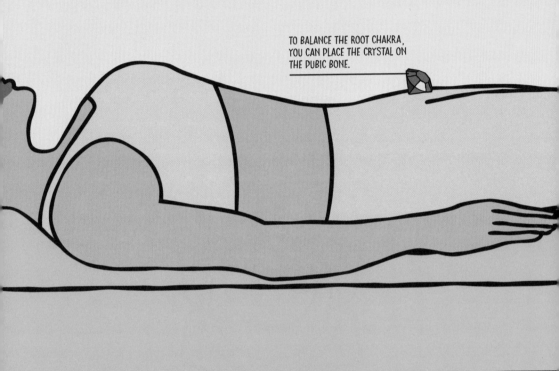

FREQUENCY

Keep the crystal on the root chakra
location and continue the meditation
for 3–5 minutes.

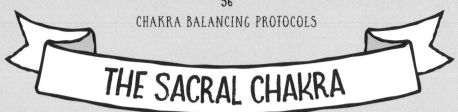

THE SACRAL CHAKRA

The sacral chakra is the second of the seven chakras and the second **physical chakra**. It is the seat of creativity in your chakra system. It governs your feelings of **pleasure** and **physical love** and sexuality. It is located just below the navel at the center of the lower abdomen, in front of the sacrum. It is connected to the element of **water** and symbolizes the fluid and **flowing** nature of life. This chakra has an energetic color of **orange** and is symbolized by the six-petaled lotus.

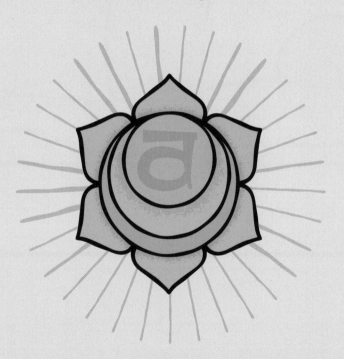

The sacral chakra is where creative energy flows to create and maintain healthy physical relationships through **physical touch**. This energy center drives your will to create and your ability to move with the changes of the world around you. When properly developed you go with the **flow of life** and easily create material abundance and feelings of **pleasure** and **joy**.

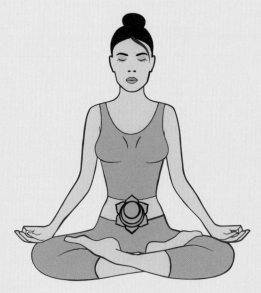

With an unbalanced sacral chakra

Imbalances in the second chakra may leave you feeling guilty or **shameful**, particularly in the area of sexuality. Sexual abuse or trauma may result in internalized anger that leaves you with **blocked feelings** and emotions. Relationships may be unstable and unbalanced, and you may be unable to allow the flow of abundance and success. **Self-sabotage** and self-criticism prevent you from moving forward in life and you blame yourself for not doing so.

If your sacral chakra is **overactive** you may experience **sexual compulsions** or **addictions**. You may be jealous or possessive in your relationships or move from one physical relationship to the next without regard to an emotional connection. You seek even more physical pleasure to overcome your feelings of guilt and frustration.

If the sacral chakra is **underactive** you may feel **shutdown** and stiff or even frigid in your sexual relationships. Issues of **impotence** or **infertility** may arise, as well as physical diseases of the pelvis. Depression and internalized shame may keep you from enjoying sexual relationships at all. You may be numb and unable to feel happiness and joy as a result of past or ongoing sexual abuse or trauma.

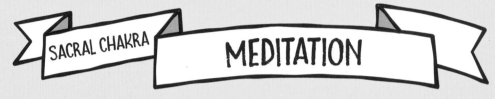

SACRAL CHAKRA — **MEDITATION**

Take long, deep breaths and, using your mind's eye, visualize chakra balancing energy spinning at the **center** of your **pelvis**. "See" the **color orange** spinning just below your navel. Allow this energy to flow freely with **joy** and respect for your gift of **creation**. Recite the following:

My sacral chakra is my second energy center and it functions to stimulate my child-like emotions and adventure.

This is the source of my creativity and inspiration.

My sexual desire and passion are born here.

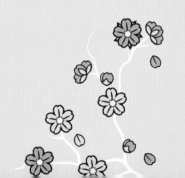

With a balanced sacral chakra

I AM EXCITED AND JOYFUL.

★

I AM FILLED WITH WONDER AND CURIOSITY.

★

I AM INSPIRED AND OPEN TO NEW EXPERIENCES.

★

I AM ENJOYING MY LIFE AND EAT GOOD FOOD.

★

I AM ALLOWING MY CREATIVE ABILITIES TO THRIVE.

★

I AM PASSIONATE AND MOTIVATED TO CREATE HAPPINESS.

★

I AM COMFORTABLE IN SOCIAL AND INTIMATE SITUATIONS.

★

MY SACRAL CHAKRA IS BALANCED AND VITAL. I AM
COMFORTABLE AND READY TO ENGAGE MY THIRD ENERGY
CENTER, THE SOLAR PLEXUS CHAKRA.

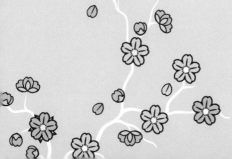

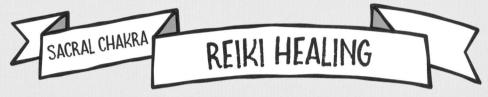

SACRAL CHAKRA

REIKI HEALING

Use the sacral chakra meditation and visualize the Reiki Universal
Life Energy flowing as you hold these hand positions.

Navel

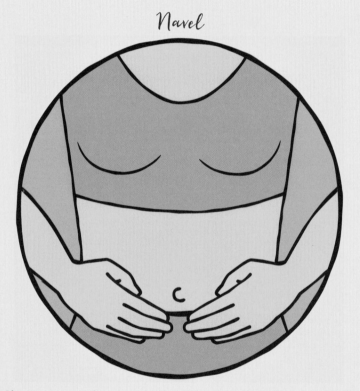

Close your eyes and cup your hands. With your palms facing you and your
fingertips pointing toward each other, place your hands on your middle abdomen.
Gently press your hands just below the navel.

FREQUENCY

Hold each hand position and continue the meditation for 2–3 minutes

See also

**WHAT IS REIKI SUBTLE
ENERGY HEALING?**
PAGES 36–37

SACRAL CHAKRA MEDITATION
PAGES 58–59

Waist

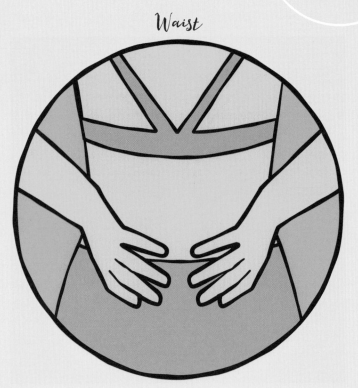

Close your eyes and cup your hands. With your palms facing you and your fingertips pointing toward each other, place your hands behind you, on the lower part of your back. Gently press the base of your palms on your waist.

SACRAL CHAKRA

FOOT REFLEXOLOGY

The reflex point for the sacral chakra is on the **inside edge** of the foot, **between** the **heel** and the **arch**. Use the sacral chakra meditation and send balancing energy to the chakra's energy center as you reflex the point.

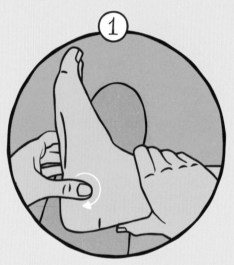

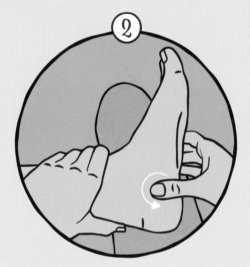

Place your right foot on your left knee. With either hand use the thumb or finger roll on the reflex point on the inside edge of the foot. Use the techniques individually or in combination.

Place your left foot on your right knee and repeat the foot reflexology technique on the reflex point between the heel and the arch of the left foot.

FREQUENCY

Flex each reflex point and continue the meditation for 2–3 minutes for each foot.

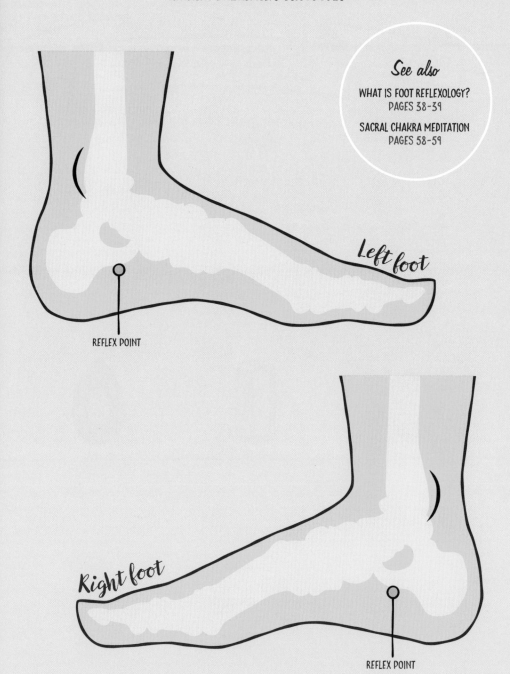

See also

WHAT IS FOOT REFLEXOLOGY?
PAGES 38-39

SACRAL CHAKRA MEDITATION
PAGES 58-59

Left foot

REFLEX POINT

Right foot

REFLEX POINT

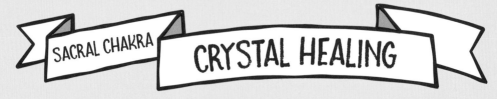

SACRAL CHAKRA

CRYSTAL HEALING

Place your chosen crystal on the sacral chakra location just below the navel—you can also simply hold the crystal in your left hand. Use the sacral chakra meditation to send healing energy from the crystal to the sacral chakra energy center.

Selection process

Choose a crystal corresponding to the sacral chakra.

CARNELIAN

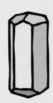

ORANGE CALCITE

SUNSTONE

See also

WHAT IS CRYSTAL
HEALING ENERGY?
PAGES 40-41

SACRAL CHAKRA MEDITATION
PAGES 58-59

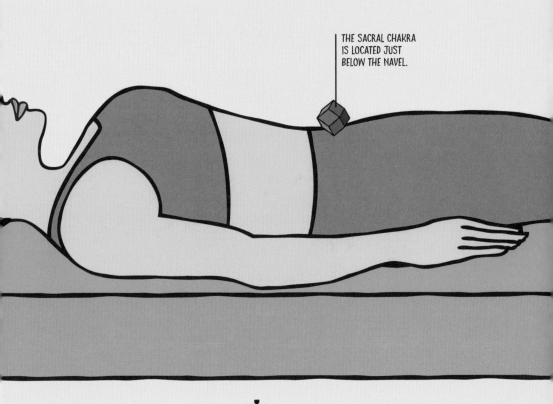

THE SACRAL CHAKRA IS LOCATED JUST BELOW THE NAVEL.

FREQUENCY

Keep the crystal on the sacral chakra location and continue the meditation for 3–5 minutes.

THE SOLAR PLEXUS CHAKRA

The solar plexus chakra is the third of the seven chakras and the third **physical chakra**. It is the core of your **personal power** in your chakra system. It governs your **self-esteem**, self-acceptance, and **self-reliance**. It is located above the navel, at the center of the upper abdomen, just below your diaphragm. It is connected to the element of fire and symbolizes the heat and energy needed to facilitate **transformation** in your life. This chakra has an energetic color of **yellow** and is symbolized by the ten-petaled lotus.

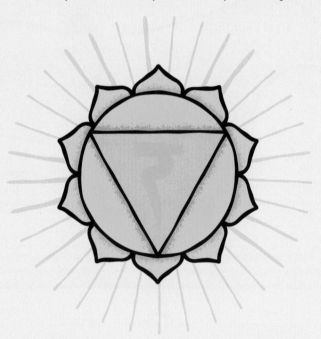

The solar plexus chakra is where the heat needed to transform your food into **fuel** and energy is generated. This energy is used by your body to accomplish everyday maintenance and **healing**, and to accommodate **change**. It is your energetic core and drives your will to **take action**. It enables your inner warrior to propel you forward to **overcome challenges** and to balance your actions with tolerance and acceptance of others.

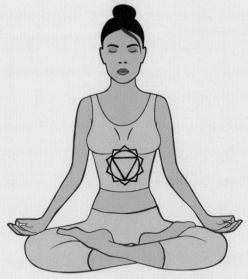

With an unbalanced solar plexus chakra

Imbalances in the third chakra may leave you filled with doubt, **self-hatred**, and **inadequacy**. These feelings may affect your ability to take charge and make decisions. Because of your lack of self-respect, you may give away your power and be left with internalized anger and resentment. This may lead to insensitivity to others. You may move through the world with **extreme responses** to minor annoyances.

If your solar plexus chakra is **overactive** you may experience **violent outbursts** and an intolerance of others, and even **bullying**. You may **blame others** for your mistakes and have a difficult time taking responsibility for your actions. An exaggerated sense of self may leave you with a need to look good and be right about everything. You may use your vanity and need for prestige to overpower and control those around you.

If the solar plexus chakra is **underactive** you may feel intimidated and **victimized** by the world. Your poor self-image may leave you paralyzed and **unable to take action**. The heat or "fire" generated by your solar plexus may be insufficient to sustain you with the energy needed to create a life you love. Your **lack of confidence** and self-doubt may leave you with a diminished sense of self, which may lead to feelings of worthlessness and wanting to withdraw or **disconnect** from the world.

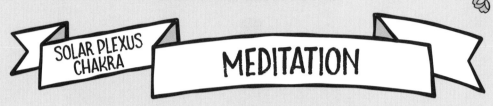

SOLAR PLEXUS CHAKRA

MEDITATION

Take long, deep breaths and, using your mind's eye, visualize chakra balancing energy spinning at the **core** of your **upper abdomen**. "See" the **color yellow** spinning below your sternum and just above your navel. Allow this energy to strengthen your **resolve** and **personal power**. Recite the following:

My solar plexus chakra is my third energy center and it functions to provide me with focus and power.

This is my source of confidence and self-esteem.

My "gut" feelings are sensed here.

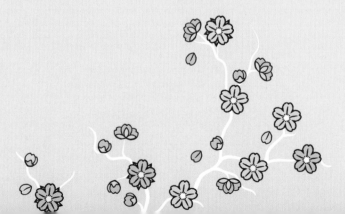

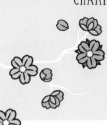

With a balanced solar plexus chakra

I AM ABLE TO CHOOSE POWERFULLY.

★

I AM CONFIDENT IN HOW I MOVE IN THE WORLD.

★

I AM SELF-AWARE AND MAKE DECISIONS WITHOUT HESITATION.

★

I AM IN CONTROL OF MY LIFE.

★

I AM ABLE TO ACT UNDER PRESSURE.

★

I AM ABLE TO ACCEPT FEEDBACK AS CONSTRUCTIVE CRITICISM.

★

MY SOLAR PLEXUS CHAKRA IS BALANCED AND VITAL. I AM
COMFORTABLE AND READY TO ENGAGE MY FOURTH ENERGY
CENTER, THE HEART CHAKRA.

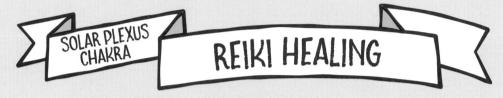

SOLAR PLEXUS CHAKRA

REIKI HEALING

Use the solar plexus chakra meditation and visualize the Reiki Universal Life Energy flowing as you hold these hand positions.

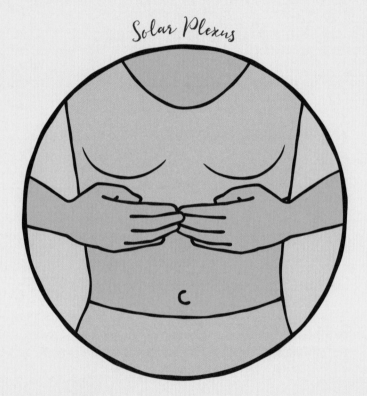

Solar Plexus

Close your eyes and cup your hands. With your palms facing you and the tips of your middle fingers touching, place your hands on your upper abdomen. Gently press your palms on the bottom of your rib cage.

FREQUENCY

Hold each hand position and continue the meditation for 2–3 minutes.

See also

**WHAT IS REIKI SUBTLE
ENERGY HEALING?
PAGES 36–37**

**SOLAR PLEXUS
CHAKRA MEDITATION
PAGES 68–69**

Ribs

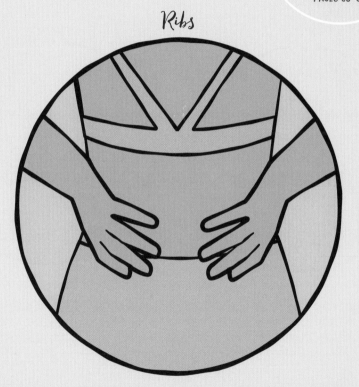

Close your eyes and cup your hands. With your palms facing you and your
fingertips pointing toward each other, place your hands behind you, on the middle
part of your back. Gently press your palms on the bottom of your rib cage.

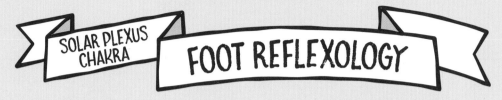

SOLAR PLEXUS CHAKRA — FOOT REFLEXOLOGY

The reflex point for the solar plexus chakra is on the **arch** on the **inside edge** of the foot. Use the solar plexus chakra meditation and send balancing energy to the chakra's energy center as you reflex the point.

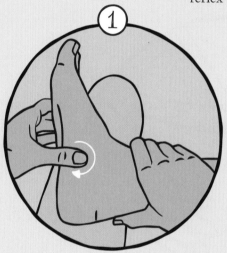

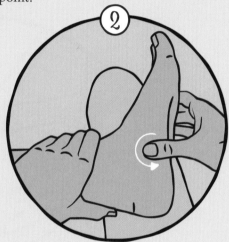

Place your right foot on your left knee. With your right or left hand use the thumb or finger roll on the reflex point on the inside edge of the arch of the foot. Use the techniques individually or in combination.

Place your left foot on your right knee and repeat the foot reflexology technique using the reflex point on the arch of the left foot.

FREQUENCY

Flex each reflex point and continue the meditation for 2–3 minutes for each foot.

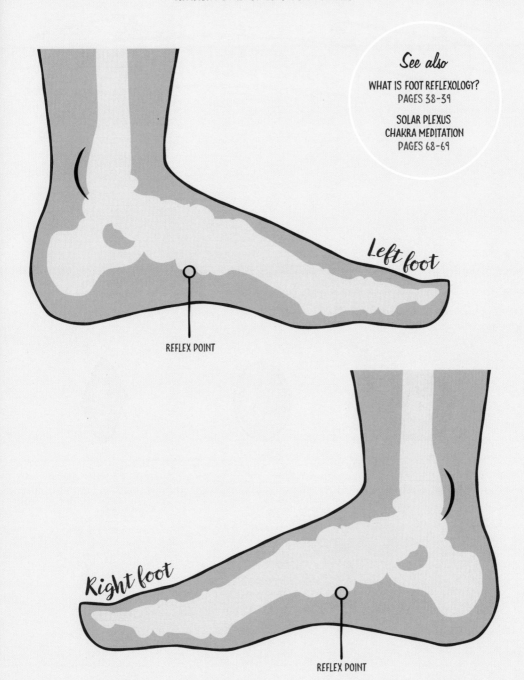

See also

WHAT IS FOOT REFLEXOLOGY?
PAGES 38-39

SOLAR PLEXUS
CHAKRA MEDITATION
PAGES 68-69

Left foot

REFLEX POINT

Right foot

REFLEX POINT

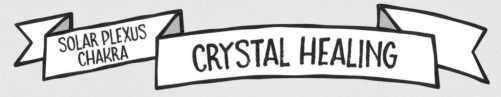

SOLAR PLEXUS CHAKRA

CRYSTAL HEALING

Place your chosen crystal on the solar plexus chakra location just above the navel—you can also simply hold the crystal in your left hand. Use the solar plexus chakra meditation to send healing energy from the crystal to the solar plexus chakra energy center.

Selection process

Choose a crystal corresponding to the solar plexus chakra.

CITRINE

YELLOW JASPER

TOPAZ

See also

WHAT IS CRYSTAL
HEALING ENERGY?
PAGES 40-41

SOLAR PLEXUS CHAKRA
MEDITATION
PAGES 68-69

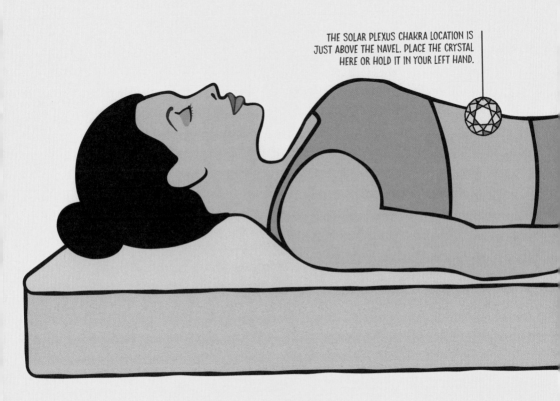

THE SOLAR PLEXUS CHAKRA LOCATION IS JUST ABOVE THE NAVEL. PLACE THE CRYSTAL HERE OR HOLD IT IN YOUR LEFT HAND.

FREQUENCY

Keep the crystal on the solar plexus chakra location and continue the meditation for 3–5 minutes.

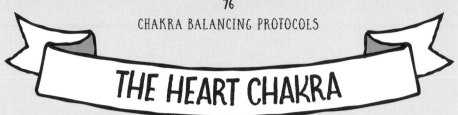

THE HEART CHAKRA

The heart chakra is the **fourth** of the seven chakras and **connects** the three **physical chakras** with the three **spriritual chakras**. It is the gateway to your **spiritual connection** to the divine. The heart chakra is located at the center of your chest between your sternum and your spine. It is connected to the element of **air** and symbolizes the highest vibration in the **physical realm**. This chakra has an energetic color of **green** and is symbolized by the 12-petaled lotus.

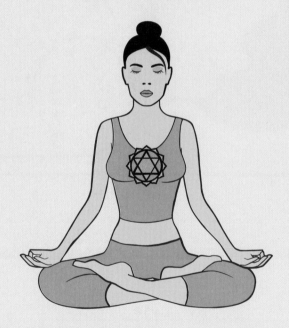

The heart chakra is where the **love** you have for yourself and others is generated. You are connected to yourself in a deep way. This energy center is the source of your ability to love and be loved. It bridges the connection to the lower three chakras and keeps you grounded and **connected** to your **higher self**. When properly developed, you are motivated by love and are able to generate **joy**, **compassion**, and empathy in your life. You easily see the **beauty** in yourself and others.

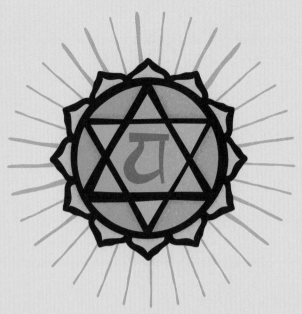

With an unbalanced heart chakra

Imbalances in the fourth chakra may leave you **disconnected** from yourself and others. You may have feelings of unprocessed **grief** or sorrow that leave you depressed or lonely. This may leave you resentful and angry, and make **relationships** very **challenging**. You may give love where it is not deserved or wanted.

If your heart chakra is **overactive** you may exhibit **codependent** tendencies and be easily hurt by the actions of others. You may consider the needs of others ahead of your own and may take on their emotions or problems. This may result in a misguided sense of what love is and lead you to be **overly affectionate** and smother your partner or your children with what you think is love. You may respond with passive-aggressive behavior, or by being **overly critical** of others.

If your heart chakra is **underactive** you may find it hard to **engage** in a romantic relationship. Because of your lack of self-love you may be unable to experience the deep connection needed to cultivate and maintain a love relationship. Unable to trust others, you may **shut down** emotionally and question your own worthiness and desire to live a life filled with joy and satisfaction.

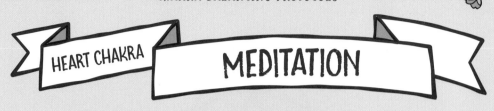

HEART CHAKRA · **MEDITATION**

Take long, deep breaths and, using your mind's eye, visualize chakra balancing energy spinning at the **center** of your **chest**. "See" the **color green** spinning between your sternum and your spine. Allow this energy to **open your heart** and generate a feeling of being **connected to others**. Recite the following:

My heart chakra is my fourth energy center and it functions to provide me with empathy and compassion toward others.

It is the source of my ability to heal myself and others and to send and receive love.

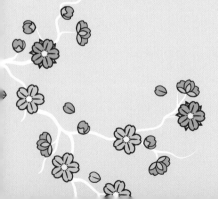

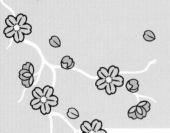

With a balanced heart chakra

I AM OPEN AND GENTLE WITH MYSELF AND OTHERS.

★

I AM SELF-LOVING AND HONOR MY DESIRES AND NEEDS.

★

I AM COMFORTABLE IN INTIMATE RELATIONSHIPS.

★

I AM LOVING, CARING, AND UNDERSTANDING.

★

I AM CONNECTED TO OTHERS.

★

I AM JOYFUL AND ABLE TO FORGIVE MYSELF AND OTHERS.

★

I AM PEACEFUL, KIND, AND COMPASSIONATE.

★

MY HEART CHAKRA IS BALANCED AND VITAL. I VALUE MYSELF
AND I AM READY TO ENGAGE MY FIFTH ENERGY CENTER,
THE THROAT CHAKRA.

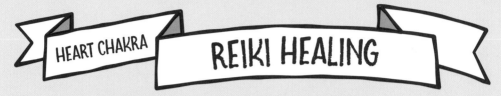

HEART CHAKRA

REIKI HEALING

Recite the heart chakra meditation and visualize the Reiki Universal Life Energy flowing as you hold these hand positions.

Heart

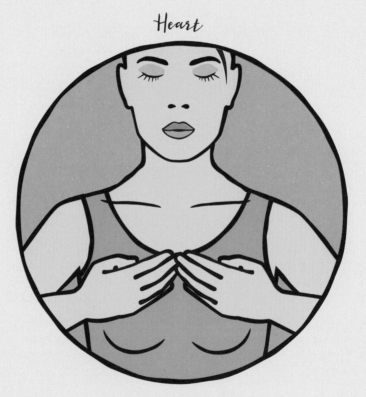

Close your eyes and cup your hands. With your palms facing you and the tips of your middle fingers touching, place your hands on your chest. Press gently on the middle part of your sternum.

FREQUENCY

Hold each hand position and continue the meditation for 2–3 minutes.

See also

WHAT IS REIKI SUBTLE
ENERGY HEALING?
PAGES 36–37

HEART CHAKRA MEDITATION
PAGES 78–79

Shoulders

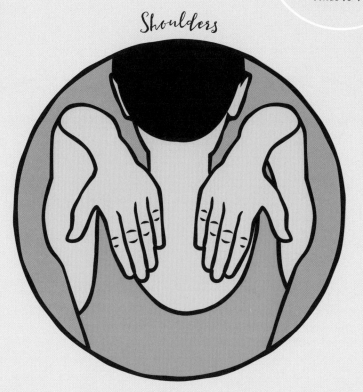

Close your eyes. Place your hands behind you, on the middle part of your shoulders, with your fingertips facing downward and inward, toward your spine. Gently press your fingers on your shoulders.

HEART CHAKRA FOOT REFLEXOLOGY

The reflex point for the heart chakra is on the **inside edge** of the foot at the **midpoint** of the **metatarsal** bone **between** the **arch** and the **base** of the **big toe**. Use the heart chakra meditation and send balancing energy to the heart chakra's energy center as you reflex the point.

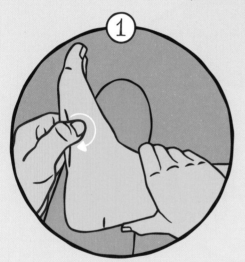

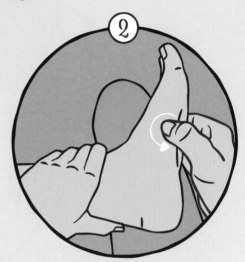

Place your right foot on your left knee. With your right or left hand use the thumb or finger roll on the reflex point on the inside edge between the arch and the base of the big toe. Use the techniques individually or in combination.

Place your left foot on your right knee and repeat the foot reflexology technique using the reflex point on the inside edge between the arch and the base of the big toe of the left foot.

FREQUENCY

Flex each reflex point and continue the meditation for 2–3 minutes for each foot.

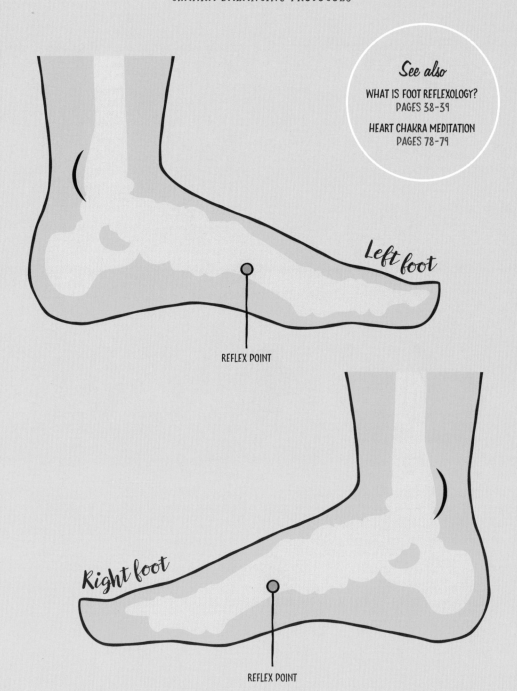

See also

WHAT IS FOOT REFLEXOLOGY?
PAGES 38-39

HEART CHAKRA MEDITATION
PAGES 78-79

Left foot

REFLEX POINT

Right foot

REFLEX POINT

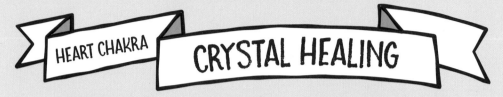

HEART CHAKRA **CRYSTAL HEALING**

Place your chosen crystal on the heart chakra location at the center of your chest—you can also simply hold the crystal in your left hand. Use the heart chakra meditation to send crystal healing energy from the crystal to the heart chakra energy center.

Selection process

Choose a crystal corresponding to the heart chakra.

ROSE QUARTZ

JADE

GREEN CALCITE

See also

WHAT IS CRYSTAL
HEALING ENERGY?
PAGES 60-61

HEART CHAKRA
MEDITATION
PAGES 78-79

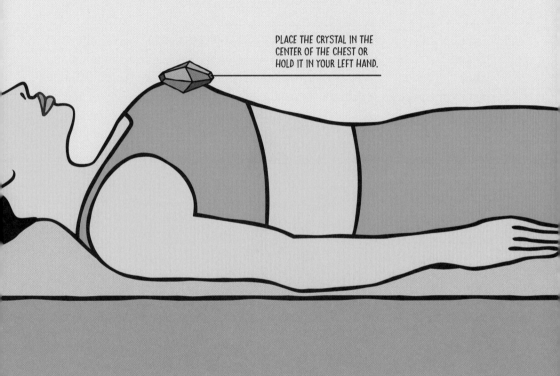

PLACE THE CRYSTAL IN THE CENTER OF THE CHEST OR HOLD IT IN YOUR LEFT HAND.

FREQUENCY

Keep the crystal on the heart chakra location and continue the meditation for 3–5 minutes.

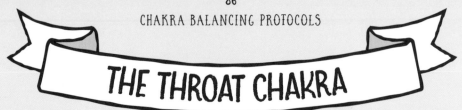

THE THROAT CHAKRA

The throat chakra is the fifth of the seven chakras and the first **spiritual chakra**. It is the energetic source of your "voice" and governs your ability to share yourself with the world. The chakra is located in the center of your neck, between your throat and your spine. It is connected to the element **ether** and translates your feelings and **emotions** into **words**. This chakra has an energetic color of **light blue** and is symbolized by the 16-petaled lotus.

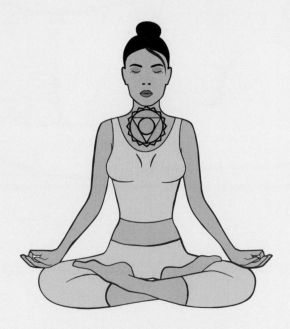

The throat chakra is the source of your **self-expression**. This energy center provides you with the power of **communication**. It functions to **connect** and balance the thoughts of the **mind** with the feelings of the heart. It assists in your ability to know when to speak and when to listen. When you share your thoughts and feelings with others, you are able to create a life you love. Your truth and **authenticity** are revealed as you share and inspire others.

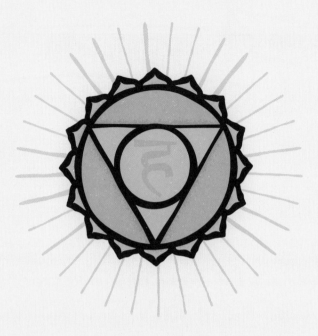

With an unbalanced throat chakra

Imbalances in the fifth chakra may leave you **reluctant** or unable to
speak your truth. You may also make things up to avoid having to
tell the truth. If you were told to be "seen and not heard" you may be
left feeling shutdown and **silenced**, and unable to express yourself.
The resulting anxiety may leave you feeling isolated and unseen.

If your throat chakra is **overactive** you may **speak before thinking**.
You may get very creative in trying to deceive others and believe that
you're telling the truth as long as you are not lying. You may be **loud**
and **insistent**, and find it very hard to stop and listen, and instead
speak nonstop about trivial matters. Gossiping and being a know-it-all
may be prevalent. Silence in a conversation may be unbearable.

If your throat chakra is **underactive** you may be **extremely shy**,
petrified to speak in public, and unable to have a one-on-one
conversation. You want to share an idea, but just cannot conjure up
the nerve to speak. When you do speak, you may be unsure and timid,
and unable to communicate your thoughts, ideas, or feelings
effectively. You end up feeing **misunderstood** and **unheard**.

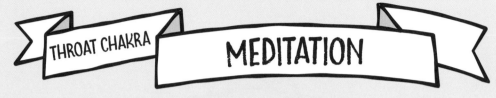

THROAT CHAKRA

MEDITATION

Take long, deep breaths and, using your mind's eye, visualize chakra balancing energy spinning at the center of your neck. "See" the **color light blue** spinning between your throat and your spine. Allow this energy to give you the ability to fully express yourself with clarity and confidence. Recite the following:

My throat chakra is my fifth energy center and it functions to provide me with the ability to powerfully communicate with others.

It is the source of my self-expression and allows me to share my gifts with the world.

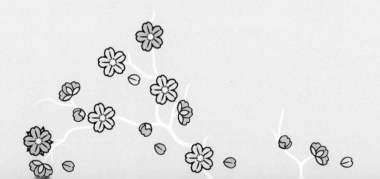

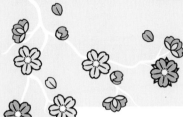

With a balanced throat chakra

I AM CONFIDENT AND CLEAR IN MY COMMUNICATIONS.

★

I AM THOUGHTFUL AND UNDERSTAND OTHERS.

★

I AM FULLY SELF-EXPRESSED AND AM SEEN IN THE WORLD.

★

I AM ABLE TO SPEAK MY AUTHENTIC TRUTH.

★

I AM ABLE TO USE MY VOICE TO CREATE AND INSPIRE OTHERS.

★

I AM ABLE TO USE A VOICE THAT IS STRONG AND VIBRANT.

★

MY THROAT CHAKRA IS BALANCED AND VITAL. I FEEL
UNDERSTOOD AND HEARD, AND I AM READY TO ENGAGE MY
SIXTH ENERGY CENTER, THE THIRD-EYE CHAKRA.

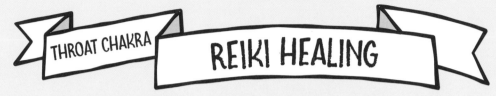

THROAT CHAKRA — REIKI HEALING

Use the throat chakra meditation and visualize the Reiki Universal
Life Energy flowing as you hold these hand positions.

Throat

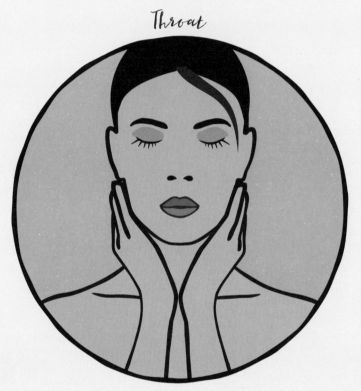

Close your eyes and cup your hands. Place your hands at the front of your throat,
with the base of your palms touching. Hover your hands beneath your jaw.

FREQUENCY

Hold each hand position and continue the meditation for 2–3 minutes.

See also

WHAT IS REIKI SUBTLE
ENERGY HEALING?
PAGES 36-37

THROAT CHAKRA MEDITATION
PAGES 88-89

Skull

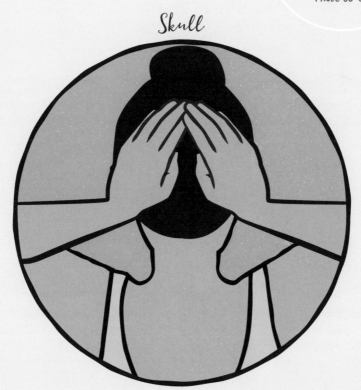

Close your eyes and place your hands on the back of your skull. Touch your
index and middle fingers together. Hover your hands over the back and
lower part of your skull.

THROAT CHAKRA — FOOT REFLEXOLOGY

The reflex point for the throat chakra is on the **inside edge** of the
foot at the **end** of the **metatarsal** bone near the **base** of the **big toe**.
Use the throat chakra meditation and send balancing energy to the
throat chakra's energy center as you reflex the point.

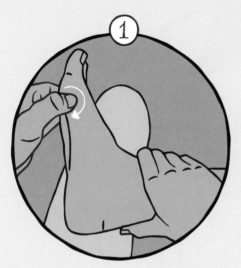

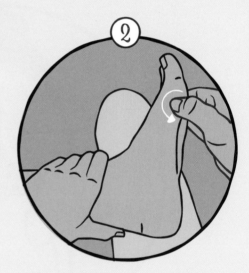

Place your right foot on your left knee. With
your right or left hand use the thumb or
finger roll on the reflex point on the inside
edge at the end of the metatarsal bone near
the base of the big toe. Use the techniques
individually or in combination.

Place your left foot on your right knee
and repeat the foot reflexology technique
using the reflex point on the inside edge
at the end of the metatarsal bone near the
base of the big toe.

FREQUENCY

Flex each reflex point and continue the
meditation for 2–3 minutes for each foot.

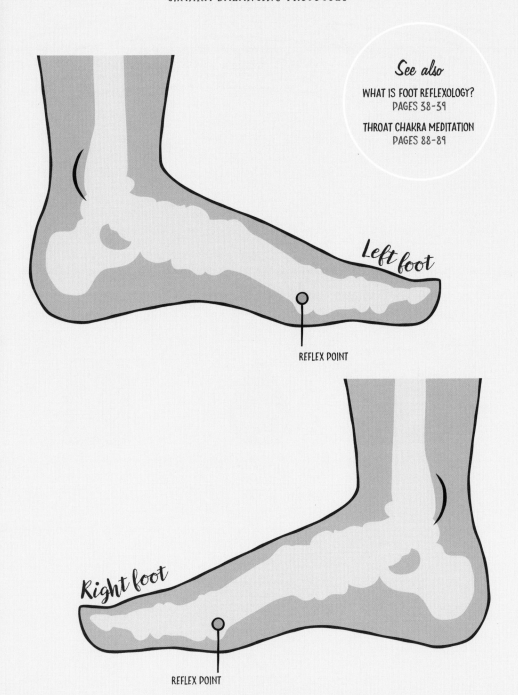

See also

WHAT IS FOOT REFLEXOLOGY?
PAGES 38–39

THROAT CHAKRA MEDITATION
PAGES 88–89

Left foot

REFLEX POINT

Right foot

REFLEX POINT

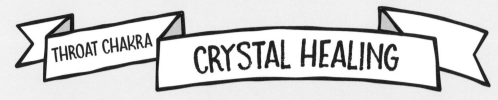

THROAT CHAKRA

CRYSTAL HEALING

Place your chosen crystal on the throat chakra location at the base of your throat—you can also simply hold the crystal in your left hand. Use the throat chakra meditation to send crystal healing energy from the crystal to the throat chakra energy center.

Selection process

Choose a crystal corresponding to the throat chakra.

AQUAMARINE

LAPIS LAZULI

TURQUOISE

See also

WHAT IS CRYSTAL
HEALING ENERGY?
PAGES 40-41

THROAT CHAKRA
MEDITATION
PAGES 88-89

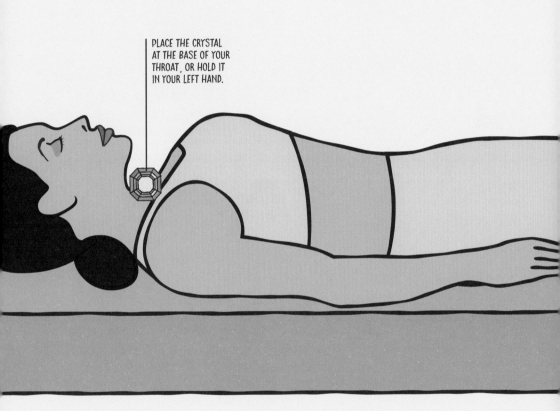

PLACE THE CRYSTAL
AT THE BASE OF YOUR
THROAT, OR HOLD IT
IN YOUR LEFT HAND.

FREQUENCY

Keep the crystal on the throat
chakra location and continue the
meditation for 3–5 minutes.

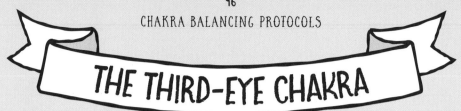

THE THIRD-EYE CHAKRA

The third-eye chakra is the sixth of the seven chakras and the second **spiritual chakra**. It is the source of your **spiritual insight** and **intuition**, and the gateway to higher consciousness. The third-eye chakra is located just above your eyebrows in the center of your forehead. It is connected to **all** of the **elements** and provides context by revealing the seen along with the unseen. This chakra has an energetic color of **indigo** and is symbolized by two petals on each side of a central circle—each petal containing the power of the 48 petals of the first five chakras, representing a 96-petaled lotus.

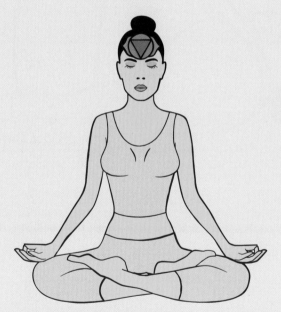

The third-eye chakra is **beyond** the **physical world**. This energy center provides you with the ability to be introspective. It functions to reveal your **highest truth** and leads you to **trust** in yourself. It provides you with the ability to see the context of situations and develop your emotional intelligence. When properly developed you have a higher overall **perspective** and are able to more keenly consider your options and choose powerfully.

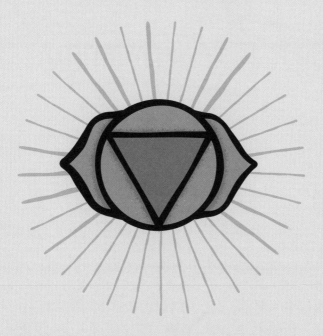

With an unbalanced third-eye chakra

Imbalances in the sixth chakra may leave you **narrow-minded** and unable to make decisions because of a **lack of clarity**. You may ignore information that is in plain sight and be unable to focus on your goal. You may appear **confused** or out-of-it to others, without realizing it yourself. Your lack of self-knowledge compromises your ability to empathize with others.

If your third-eye chakra is **overactive** you may have nightmares, visions, or psychic disturbances. You may suffer from delusions and move through the world always in your head, and have difficulty grounding yourself. Being lost in your thoughts, you may be unable to connect with others in a deep and meaningful way.

If your third-eye chakra is **underactive** you may have trouble trusting your intuition. Poor memory and **disorientation** may leave you unable to see the path you are on or the direction you are going in life. Rather than learning from your experiences, you may repeat the **same mistakes** over and over, expecting a different result.

THIRD-EYE CHAKRA · MEDITATION

Take long, deep breaths and, using your mind's eye, visualize chakra balancing energy spinning between your **eyebrows** at the **base** of your **forehead**. "See" the **color indigo** spinning behind your eyebrows at the center of your head. Allow this energy to provide you with the ability to see **beyond the physical** and trust your **intuition**. Recite the following:

My third-eye chakra is my sixth energy center and it functions to provide me with insight and intuition.

It is the source of my "sixth sense" and allows me to see myself and others as we really are.

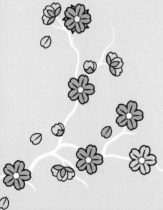

With a balanced third-eye chakra

I AM INTUITIVE AND SEE THE UNSEEN.

★

I AM AWARE AND TRUST WHAT I SEE.

★

I AM BLISSFUL IN MY VISIONS AND SEE THE BIG PICTURE.

★

I AM RATIONAL AND INSIGHTFUL IN MY THINKING.

★

I AM IMAGINATIVE AND CREATIVE.

★

I AM DISCIPLINED AND ABLE TO CONCENTRATE AND DIRECT MY ATTENTION.

★

I AM SELF-REFLECTIVE AND KNOW WHO I AM.

★

MY THIRD-EYE CHAKRA IS BALANCED AND VITAL. I REMAIN FLEXIBLE AND SEE THE HIGH GROUND, AND I AM READY TO ENGAGE MY SEVENTH ENERGY CENTER, THE CROWN CHAKRA.

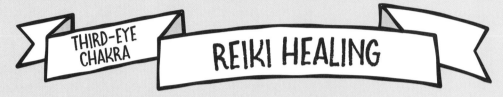

THIRD-EYE CHAKRA · REIKI HEALING

Use the third-eye chakra meditation and visualize the Reiki
Universal Life Energy flowing as you hold these hand positions.

Eyes

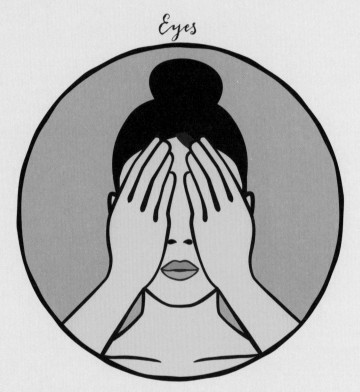

Close your eyes and cup your hands. Hover your hands over your eyes.
With your fingertips, lightly touch the top of your forehead.

FREQUENCY

Hold each hand position and continue the meditation for 2–3 minutes.

See also

WHAT IS REIKI SUBTLE ENERGY HEALING?
PAGES 36-37

THIRD-EYE CHAKRA MEDITATION
PAGES 98-99

Temples

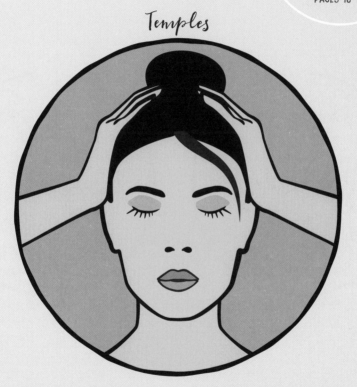

Close your eyes and cup your hands. Hover your hands over your temples/ears.
With your fingertips, lightly touch the top of your head.

THIRD-EYE CHAKRA

FOOT REFLEXOLOGY

The reflex point for the third-eye chakra is on the **inside edge** of the foot at the **first joint** of the **big toe**. Use the third-eye chakra meditation and send balancing energy to the third-eye chakra's energy center as you reflex the point.

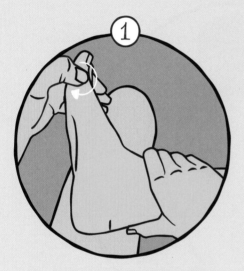

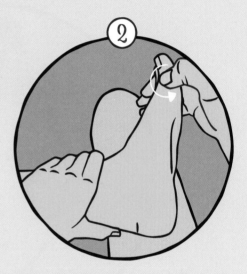

Place your right foot on your left knee. With your right or left hand use the thumb or finger roll on the reflex point on the inside edge of the foot at the first joint of the big toe. Use the techniques individually or in combination.

Place your left foot on your right knee and repeat the foot reflexology technique using the reflex point on the inside edge of the foot at the first joint of the big toe.

FREQUENCY

Flex each reflex point and continue the meditation for 2–3 minutes for each foot.

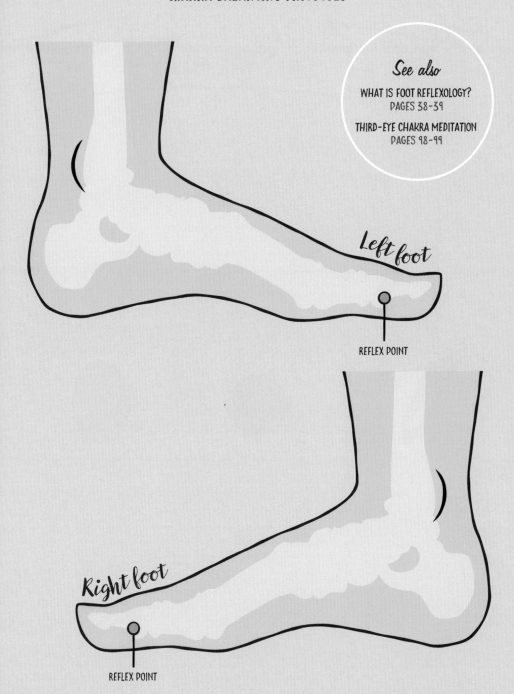

See also

WHAT IS FOOT REFLEXOLOGY?
PAGES 38-39

THIRD-EYE CHAKRA MEDITATION
PAGES 98-99

Left foot

REFLEX POINT

Right foot

REFLEX POINT

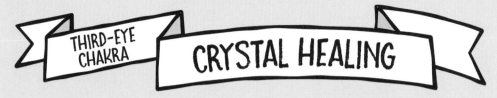

THIRD-EYE CHAKRA

CRYSTAL HEALING

Place your chosen crystal on the third-eye chakra location at the bottom of the forehead between the eyebrows—you can also simply hold the crystal in your left hand. Use the third-eye chakra meditation to send crystal healing energy from the crystal to the third-eye chakra energy center.

Selection process

Choose a crystal corresponding to the third-eye chakra.

AMETHYST

PURPLE FLUORITE

LEPIDOLITE

See also

WHAT IS CRYSTAL
HEALING ENERGY?
PAGES 40-41

THIRD-EYE CHAKRA
MEDITATION
PAGES 98-99

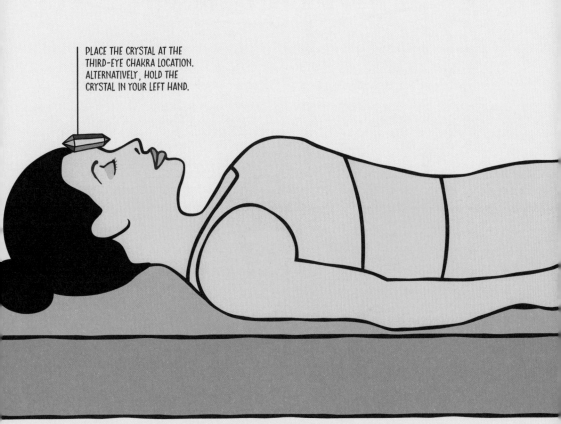

PLACE THE CRYSTAL AT THE
THIRD-EYE CHAKRA LOCATION.
ALTERNATIVELY, HOLD THE
CRYSTAL IN YOUR LEFT HAND.

FREQUENCY

Keep the crystal on the third-eye
chakra location and continue the
meditation for 3–5 minutes.

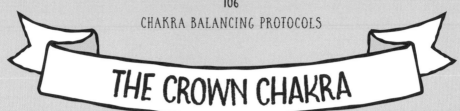

THE CROWN CHAKRA

The crown chakra is the seventh of the seven chakras and the third **spiritual chakra**. It is your direct **connection** to your **higher self** and the divine. The crown chakra is located at the top and center of your head. It is connected to **all** of the **elements** and allows you to experience the oneness of the universe. This chakra has an energetic color of **violet** or white and is symbolized by a thousand-petaled lotus.

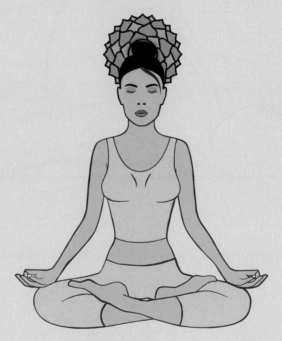

The crown chakra is connected to the realm of the **infinite** and timeless. This energy center provides the opportunity to experience the highest forms of **consciousness**. It functions to allow feelings of joy and **bliss**, peace and **transcendence**, and enables you to experience the mystical aspects of life. When properly developed you are able to know and understand the temporary nature of all things and the eternal nature of individual consciousness within the source of all that is.

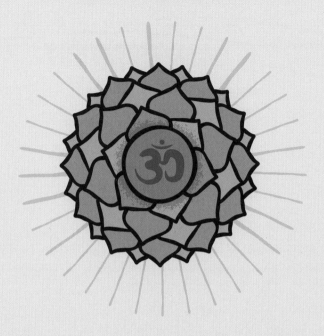

With an unbalanced crown chakra

Imbalances in the seventh chakra may leave you **disconnected** from any sort of **spiritual** reality. You may move from one type of religion to another searching for answers to spiritual questions. You may land in the "self-help merry-go-round," applying a lot of effort to make a connection to the divine, all to no avail.

If your crown chakra is **overactive** you may experience restless thinking known as the "monkey mind." Your **thoughts overtake** you and you are **unable** to connect or **engage** with those around you. You engage in materialistic behavior and may be unable to let things go. You may **hoard** things or be afraid of losing them because you are **overly attached** to them.

If your crown chakra is **underactive** you may be drawn to **extremist** religions to avoid having to take responsibility for your life. You may find it a relief being told what to do and how to do it. You may also revel in the world of intellectuals who base their experiences only on **scientific** facts and things that can be proven in the material world. All this may leave you feeling lost, **alienated**, and **spiritually disconnected**.

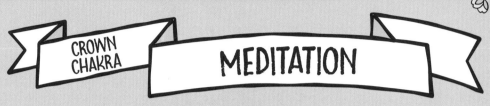

CROWN CHAKRA **MEDITATION**

Take long, deep breaths and, using your mind's eye, visualize chakra balancing energy spinning at the **top** of your **head**. "See" the **color violet** spinning between your crown and your spine. Allow this energy to provide you with the ability to experience your **divinity** and connect to your **life purpose**. Recite the following:

My crown chakra is my seventh energy center and it functions to provide me with a connection to the infinite and timeless nature of the universe.

It is the source of my oneness with the divine and allows me to have a magical sense of being.

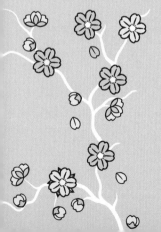

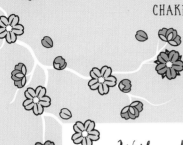

With a balanced crown chakra

I AM LIMITLESS AND CONNECTED TO MY HIGHER SELF.

★

I AM SPIRITUALLY CONNECTED TO THE DIVINE.

★

I AM ABLE TO TRANSCEND THE BOUNDARIES OF THE
PHYSICAL WORLD.

★

I AM FREE AND DISCOVER THE DIVINE MYSTERIES OF LIFE.

★

I AM BEYOND SPACE AND TIME.

★

I AM ONE WITH THE UNIVERSE AND EXPERIENCE
JOY-FILLED BLISS.

★

MY CROWN CHAKRA IS BALANCED AND VITAL. I HAVE A
SENSE OF OVERALL PEACE AND WELLNESS, AND I AM OPEN
TO INFINITE POSSIBILITIES.

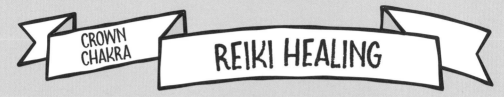

CROWN CHAKRA

REIKI HEALING

Use the crown chakra meditation and visualize the Reiki Universal Life Energy flowing as you hold these hand positions.

Eyes

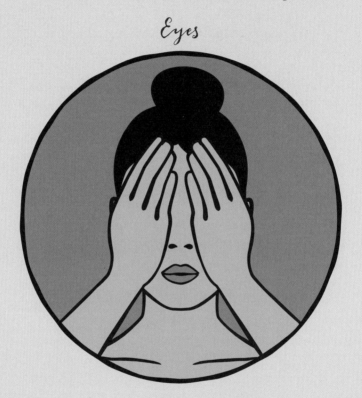

Close your eyes and cup your hands. Hover your hands over your eyes. With your fingertips, lightly touch the top of your forehead.

FREQUENCY

Hold each hand position and continue the meditation for 2–3 minutes.

See also

**WHAT IS REIKI SUBTLE
ENERGY HEALING?**
PAGES 36–37

CROWN CHAKRA MEDITATION
PAGES 108–109

Temples

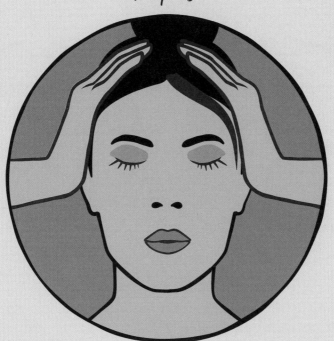

Close your eyes and cup your hands. Hover your hands over your temples/ears.
With your fingertips, lightly touch the top of your head.

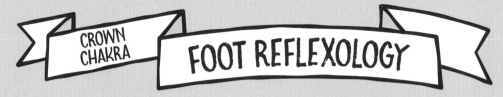

CROWN CHAKRA — FOOT REFLEXOLOGY

The reflex point for the crown chakra is on the **tip** of the **big toe**.
Use the crown chakra meditation and send balancing energy to the
crown chakra's energy center as you reflex the point.

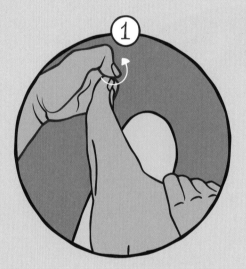

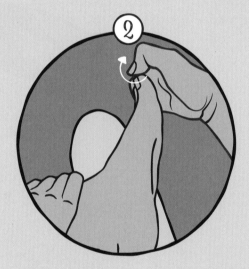

Place your right foot on your left knee. With
your right or left hand use the thumb or
finger roll on the reflex point on the tip of
the big toe. Use the techniques individually
or in combination.

Place your left foot on your right knee and
repeat the foot reflexology technique using
the reflex point on the tip of the big toe.

FREQUENCY

Flex each reflex point and continue the
meditation for 2–3 minutes for each foot.

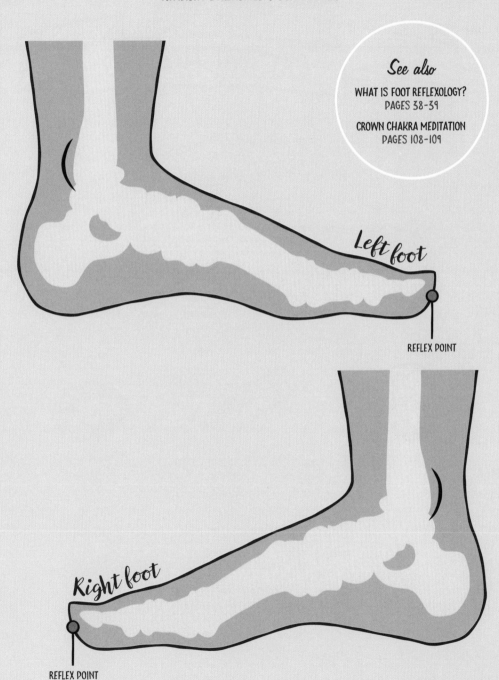

See also

WHAT IS FOOT REFLEXOLOGY?
PAGES 38-39

CROWN CHAKRA MEDITATION
PAGES 108-109

Left foot

REFLEX POINT

Right foot

REFLEX POINT

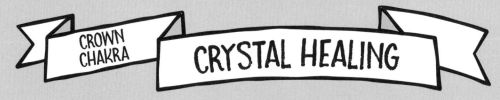

CROWN CHAKRA

CRYSTAL HEALING

Place your chosen crystal on the crown chakra location at or near the crown of your head—you can also simply hold the crystal in your left hand. Use the crown chakra meditation to send crystal healing energy from the crystal to the crown chakra energy center.

Selection process

Choose a crystal corresponding to the crown chakra.

CLEAR QUARTZ

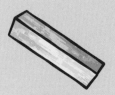

SELENITE

HERKIMER DIAMOND

See also

WHAT IS CRYSTAL
HEALING ENERGY?
PAGES 40-41

CROWN CHAKRA MEDITATION
PAGES 108-109

PLACE THE CRYSTAL
NEAR THE CROWN OF
THE HEAD, OR HOLD IT
IN YOUR LEFT HAND.

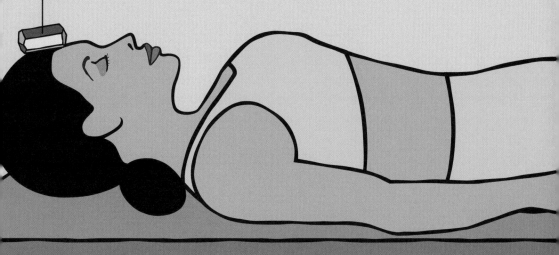

FREQUENCY

Keep the crystal on the crown
chakra location and continue the
meditation for 3–5 minutes.

RESOURCES

CHAKRA REFERENCE TABLE

This table can be used to identify which chakras to balance based on your intuition.

REFERENCE CATEGORY	ROOT	SACRAL	SOLAR PLEXUS
COLOR	Red	Orange	Yellow
LOCATION	At the base of the spine between the genitals and the anus	Slightly below the navel at the center of the lower abdomen	Slightly above the navel below the diaphragm
BODY PARTS	Colon, anus, prostate, legs, feet	Pelvic area, kidneys, urinary system, hips, reproductive organs, pelvic area	Abdomen, lower back, stomach, pancreas, spleen, liver, gallbladder, intestines, pancreas
ENDOCRINE GLAND	Adrenal	Reproductive organs	Pancreas
CRYSTALS	Shungite, tiger's eye, hematite, fire agate, black tourmaline	Citrine, carnelian, moonstone, coral	Malachite, calcite, citrine, topaz
ESSENTIAL OILS	Clove, vetiver, marjoram, myrrh	Sandalwood, patchouli, ylang ylang	Chamomile, lemon, thyme
ELEMENT	Earth	Water	Fire
ZODIAC SIGNS	Aries, Taurus, Scorpio, Capricorn	Cancer, Libra, Scorpio	Leo, Sagittarius, Virgo
PLANETS	Mars, Saturn	Moon, Venus, Mars, Mercury	Sun, Jupiter, Mars, Mercury
MINDSET	I am	I feel	I do
TONE	C	D	E
SENSE	Smell	Taste	Sight
SYMBOL	Four-petaled lotus	Six-petaled lotus	Ten-petaled lotus
MANTRA	Lam	Vam	Ram

Review the table to see what resonates with you and identify the chakras to balance. Then refer to the relevant chakra balancing protocols in Chapter 3.

CHAKRA			
HEART	**THROAT**	**THIRD-EYE**	**CROWN**
Green	Light blue	Indigo	Violet, white
Center of the chest between the sternum and the spine	At the center of the neck between the throat and the spine	Slightly above the eyebrows at the center of the forehead	At the top and center of the head
Thoracic cavity, heart, upper back, rib cage, chest, circulatory system, lungs	Mouth, jaw, ears, throat, vocal cords, neck, trachea, thyroid, shoulders, arms, hands	Eyes, nose, sinuses, pituitary, hypothalamus, medulla	Brain, pineal gland, cerebral cortex, cranium
Thymus	Thyroid	Pituitary	Pineal
Rose quartz, jade, green calcite, green tourmaline	Lapis lazuli, turquoise, aquamarine	Amethyst, purple fluorite, black obsidian	Selenite, clear quartz, amethyst, diamond
Geranium, bergamot, rose, melissa	Frankincense, neroli, sage	Lavender, jasmine, rosemary	Frankincense, peppermint, lotus
Air	Ether	All elements	All elements
Leo, Libra	Gemini, Taurus, Aquarius	Sagittarius, Aquarius, Pisces	Capricorn, Pisces
Sun, Venus, Saturn	Mars, Venus, Uranus	Mercury, Venus, Uranus	Saturn, Neptune
I love	I communicate	I see	I accept
F	G	A	B
Touch	Sound	All, plus sixth sense	Beyond senses
12-petaled lotus	16-petaled lotus	96-petaled lotus	Thousand-petaled lotus
Yam	Ham	Sham	Om

AILMENTS DIRECTORY

Use this table to identify the chakras associated with the ailments or conditions you would like to address, then refer to the relevant chakra balancing protocols in Chapter 3.

AILMENT/ISSUE	DESCRIPTION	CHAKRAS TO BALANCE
ADDICTION/ALCOHOL AND DRUG ABUSE	Addictions of all kinds are often a result of medicating pain from emotional issues.	All chakras
ADRENAL FATIGUE	Prolonged stress can cause the adrenal glands to fatigue and result in a variety of symptoms, from tiredness and feeling down to weight gain.	Root, solar plexus
ALLERGIES	The liver cleanses the blood of toxins and chemical buildup that may contribute to allergies.	Solar plexus
ANGER	Anger based on a fundamental fear for our survival when none exists can cause disease in our lives.	Root, all chakras
ANXIETY/NERVOUSNESS	Grounding yourself and relaxing the diaphragm muscle can help lower respiration and heart rates.	Root, solar plexus
ARTHRITIS	For pain and stiffness associated with arthritis, balance chakras that correspond to the affected body part.	All chakras or specific location
BACK PAIN: LOWER	For lower back pain and stiffness, it is helpful to relax the muscles attached to the lumbar spine in addition to relaxing the broader lumbar area.	Root, sacral
BACK PAIN: MIDDLE	Feeling heartbroken or unloved can be associated with middle back pain.	Solar plexus, heart

AILMENT/ISSUE	DESCRIPTION	CHAKRAS TO BALANCE
BACK PAIN: UPPER	Difficulty in expressing feelings or communicating can create tension and pain in the upper back.	Heart, throat
BRAIN AND NERVOUS SYSTEM ISSUES	Issues with the brain or nervous system can cause coordination problems, epilepsy, Parkinson's disease, mental illness, and learning disabilities.	Third-eye, crown
BREATHING ISSUES/ ASTHMA	It is important to help the lungs and bronchial tubes to relax, which may ease labored breathing.	Heart
BRONCHITIS	Bronchitis symptoms include cough, chest discomfort, and shortness of breath.	Heart, throat
CANCER	Relief from the side-effects of chemotherapy and radiation therapy. Cancer can manifest in many different places in the body.	All chakras or specific location
COLD/FLU	Helping the immune system to work more efficiently is key to getting over a cold or flu faster.	All chakras or specific location
DEPRESSION	A relaxing and soothing overall session can help provide emotional balance.	All chakras
DERMATITIS (ATOPIC)/ ECZEMA	For symptoms of itching, redness, and dry skin, balance chakras that correspond to the affected body part.	All chakras or specific location
DIABETES	In some forms of diabetes, the pancreas is not producing enough insulin, which is needed to regulate blood sugar (glucose).	Solar plexus, third-eye

AILMENT/ISSUE	DESCRIPTION	CHAKRAS TO BALANCE
DIGESTIVE ISSUES	Many digestive issues, such as diarrhea, constipation, colitis, indigestion, heartburn, acid reflux, irritable bowel syndrome, diverticulitis, gastritis, Crohn's disease, and even colorectal cancer can be related to imbalances in the solar plexus and sacral chakras.	Solar plexus, sacral
DIZZINESS/ INNER EAR ISSUES	Dizziness is often caused by imbalance of the inner ear.	Third-eye, crown
EAR INFECTION	Ear infections can be very painful.	Third-eye
EATING ISSUES/ ANOREXIA/BULIMIA	Issues with the power center may create a feeling of lack of control and lack of confidence, leading to harsh self-judgment.	Solar plexus
EYE FATIGUE	One of the most common causes of eye fatigue is staring too long at digital devices.	Third-eye
GALLSTONES	The gallbladder plays an important role in regulating cholesterol.	Solar plexus
GYNECOLOGICAL ISSUES	Issues relating to reproduction correspond to the creative energy center.	Sacral
HEADACHE	Headache pain can have a variety of causes and can be felt in different areas of the head.	Third-eye, crown
HEMORRHOIDS	Hemorrhoids are sometimes caused by constipation and can be very uncomfortable.	Root
HEPATITIS	Inflammation of the liver can lead to serious health conditions.	Solar plexus

AILMENT/ISSUE	DESCRIPTION	CHAKRAS TO BALANCE
HIATAL HERNIA	Hiatal hernia is caused by part of the stomach bulging through the diaphragm muscle.	Heart, solar plexus
HICCUPS	Hiccups are sudden spasms of the diaphragm muscle.	Solar plexus
HIGH BLOOD PRESSURE (HYPERTENSION)	It is important to relax the entire body for issues such as high blood pressure.	Solar plexus, heart
HIP PAIN	For any hip pain, balance the chakra corresponding to the affected area.	Sacral
IMPOTENCE	Impotence can result from physical or mental health issues.	Root, sacral
INGUINAL HERNIA	Inguinal hernia can cause severe pain from the weakened abdominal wall.	Root, sacral
INSOMNIA	An overactive mind that is ungrounded and nervous can cause difficulty in getting a good night's sleep.	Third-eye
JOINT PAIN (KNEE, ELBOW, OR SHOULDER)	For arthritis, bursitis, or tendonitis of the knee, elbow, or shoulder joints, balance the chakras corresponding to the affected area.	All chakras or specific location
KIDNEY STONES	Kidney stones are small, hard deposits of minerals and acid salts inside your kidneys.	Sacral, solar plexus
LEG PAIN/LEG CRAMPS	For pain from vigorous exercise, leg cramps, or leg strain, balance the chakras corresponding to the lower back.	Root, sacral

AILMENT/ISSUE	DESCRIPTION	CHAKRAS TO BALANCE
MENOPAUSE	Significant hormonal changes occur during menopause and can result in a lot of discomfort.	**All chakras**
MIGRAINES	Reducing tension in the head and neck can provide pain relief from migraines. Balance the chakras corresponding to the head and neck.	**Throat, third-eye, crown**
NAUSEA/ MORNING SICKNESS	Nausea of any kind can be helped by balancing the energy near the inner ear, the diaphragm, solar plexus, and stomach. Many women suffer from nausea in the first trimester of pregnancy.	**Solar plexus, third-eye**
NECK PAIN/STIFF NECK	To ease neck tension, pain, and stiffness it is helpful to balance the chakra corresponding to the affected area.	**Throat**
PREMENSTRUAL SYNDROME (PMS) AND MENSTRUAL CRAMPS	Premenstrual syndrome usually starts about one week before menstruation and can cause pain in the pelvis and lower abdomen.	**Sacral, throat**
PROSTATE ISSUES/ ENLARGED PROSTATE	Many men, as they age, have an enlarged prostate resulting in issues that may affect normal urination.	**Root, sacral**
PSORIASIS	Psoriasis, a chronic skin disorder, can cause itchy, red, raised, scaly patches to appear on the skin.	**All chakras or specific location**
SCIATICA	The sciatic nerve starts at the lower back and runs through the buttocks and down each leg.	**Root, sacral**
SINUS CONGESTION/ SINUSITIS	From allergies to a cold, you can find relief by balancing the chakra corresponding to the sinuses.	**Third-eye**

AILMENT/ISSUE	DESCRIPTION	CHAKRAS TO BALANCE
SORE THROAT	A sore throat is often the first sign of a cold.	Throat
STOMACH ACHE	Stomach pain can be caused by a variety of issues.	Solar plexus
TEETH/GUM ISSUES	Poor oral hygiene can cause serious systemic health issues.	Throat, third-eye
TEMPORAL MANDIBULAR JOINT (TMJ) DISORDER/ JAW TENSION	TMJ disorder can cause pain in the jaw joint and muscles in the neck and throat.	Throat, third-eye
THYROID IMBALANCES AND DYSFUNCTION	The thyroid gland is located at the base of the neck and is essential for producing hormones that affect metabolism.	Throat, third-eye
TINNITUS/RINGING OF THE EARS	Tinnitus is commonly referred to as ringing or buzzing in the ears and can be either temporary or chronic.	Third-eye
TONSILLITIS	Tonsillitis is an inflammation or infection of the tonsils at the back of the throat.	Throat
ULCER	Common symptoms of stomach ulcers are burning stomach pain, bloating, feelings of fullness, fatty food intolerance, and nausea.	Solar plexus
URINARY/BLADDER ISSUES	The inability to let go and release the stresses of life can cause difficulty with urination or leave you vulnerable to urinary tract infections.	Sacral
URINARY TRACT INFECTIONS (UTIS)	Candida, yeast, and other urinary tract infections can cause burning and be very painful.	Sacral

INDEX

A

addiction 120
adrenal fatigue 120
ailments, specific 23,
  120–125
alcohol abuse 120
allergies 120
anger 120
anorexia 122
anxiety 120
arthritis 120
asthma/breathing
  issues 121
astrology 23

B

back pain
  lower 120
  middle 120
  upper 121
balancing, chakra
  19–31
basic principles 14–19
bath, natural light 42
bath, water 43
bladder issues/urinary
  125
body parts 24–27,
  118–119
brain/nervous system
  issues 121
breathing issues/
  asthma 121
bronchitis 121
bulimia 122

C

cancer 121
centering/grounding
  18
chakras, primary 16–17
characteristics, chakra
  23
cold/flu 121
color psychology 23,
  118–119
crown chakra 16–17
  balanced 109
  crystal healing
    114–115
  emotional
    conditions 31
  endocrine gland 27
  foot reflexology
    112–113
  meditation 108
  Reference Table 119
  reiki healing
    110–111
  spiritual 106
  unbalanced 107
crystal geode cave/
  cluster 43
crystal healing energy
  33, 34–35, 40–41,
  118–119
crystals, choosing
  40–41
crystals, energizing/
  cleansing 42–43

D

depression 121
dermatitis (atopic)/
  eczema 121
diabetes 121
digestive issues 122
dizziness 122
drug abuse 120

E

ear infection 122
ear issues, inner 122
eating issues 122
eczema/dermatitis
  (atopic) 121
elbow pain 123
elements, five 23,
  118–119
emotional conditions
  28–31
endocrine glands
  25–27, 118–119
energy centers 14
enlarged prostate/
  prostate issues 124
essential oils 33,
  118–119
eye fatigue 122

F

flu/cold 121

G

gallstones 122
grounding/centering
  18
gum/teeth issues 125
gynecological issues
  122

H

headache 122
heart chakra 16–17
  balanced 79
  connecting 76
  crystal healing
    84–85
  emotional
    conditions 30
  endocrine gland 26
  foot reflexology
    82–83
  meditation 78

Reference Table 119
reiki healing 80–81
unbalanced 77
hemorrhoids 122
hepatitis 122
hernia, hiatal/inguinal
  123
hiccups 123
high blood pressure
  (hypertension) 123
hip pain 123
hypertension (high
  blood pressure) 123

I

impotence 123
insomnia 123
intention 18

J

jaw tension/temporal
  mandibular joint
  disorder 125
joint pain (knee,
  elbow, shoulder)
  123

K

kidney stones 123
knee pain 123

L

leg pain/cramps 123
location, body 118–119

M

mantras 33, 118–119
meditation 18, 33
menopause 124

menstrual cramps/
premenstrual
syndrome 124
migraines 124
mindset 118–119
modality, which 32–33
morning sickness 124
mudras 33

N
nausea/morning
sickness 124
neck pain/stiff neck
124
nervous system/brain
issues 121
nervousness 120

O
organs, physical 24–27
out-of-balance
conditions,
emotional 28–31

P
planets 118–119
pranayama 33
premenstrual
syndrome/menstrual
cramps 124
prostate issues/
enlarged prostate
124
protocols, which
34–35
psoriasis 124

R
Reference Table 23,
118–119
reflexology 33

reflexology, foot
34–35, 38–39
reiki 33, 34–35, 36–37
ringing of ears/
tinnitus 125
root chakra 16–17
balanced 49
crystal healing
54–55
emotional
conditions 28
endocrine gland 25
foot reflexology
52–53
meditation 48
physical 46–47
Reference Table 118
reiki healing 50–51
unbalanced 47

S
sacral chakra 16–17
balanced 59
crystal healing
64–65
emotional
conditions 29
endocrine gland 25
foot reflexology
62–63
meditation 58
physical 56
Reference Table 118
reiki healing 60–61
unbalanced 57
salt 43
sciatica 124
sense 118–119
shoulder pain 123
sinus congestion/
sinusitis 124
smudging 43

solar plexus chakra
16–17
balanced 69
crystal healing
74–75
emotional
conditions 29
endocrine gland 25
foot reflexology
72–73
meditation 68
physical 66
Reference Table 118
reiki healing 70–71
unbalanced 67
sore throat 125
sound therapy 23
stomach ache 125
symbol, lotus 118–119

T
teeth/gum issues 125
temporal mandibular
joint disorder/jaw
tension 125
third-eye chakra
16–17
balanced 99
crystal healing
104–105
emotional
conditions 31
endocrine gland 27
foot reflexology
102–103
meditation 98
Reference Table 119
reiki healing
100–101
spiritual 96
unbalanced 97
throat chakra 16–17
balanced 89

crystal healing
94–95
emotional
conditions 30
endocrine gland 26
foot reflexology
92–93
meditation 88
Reference Table 119
reiki healing 90–91
spiritual 86
unbalanced 87
thyroid imbalances/
dysfunction 125
tinnitus/ringing of
ears 125
tone 118–119
tonsillitis 125

U
ulcer 125
urinary/bladder issues
125
urinary tract infections
125
Usui Shiki Ryoho see
reiki

W
water bath 43
willingness 18

Y
yantras 33
yoga 33

Z
zodiac signs 118–119

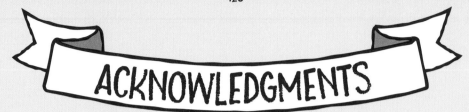

ACKNOWLEDGMENTS

IT NEVER CEASES TO AMAZE ME HOW THE UNIVERSE CONTINUES TO PROVIDE UNIMAGINABLE OPPORTUNITIES. THIS BOOK IS ONE OF THOSE OPPORTUNITIES.

FIRST AND FOREMOST, THANK YOU TO MY AMAZING PUBLISHING TEAM AT THE QUARTO GROUP FOR THEIR GUIDANCE AND SUPPORT IN CREATING A FUN, BEAUTIFUL, AND ACCESSIBLE HOW-TO BOOK. IT HAS BEEN A JOY!

I'D ALSO LIKE TO THANK MY CLIENTS AND FELLOW PRACTITIONERS FOR REMINDING ME WHY I DO WHAT I DO AND FOR INSPIRING ME TO DEEPEN MY KNOWLEDGE AND SHARE WHAT I LEARN.

FINALLY, THANK YOU TO MY HUSBAND STEVEN, FOR BELIEVING IN ME, ESPECIALLY WHEN I STRUGGLE TO BELIEVE IN MYSELF.

BE WELL.

Other books in the series

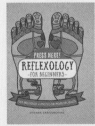
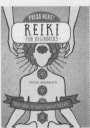
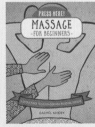
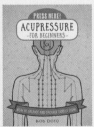
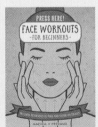

ISBN 978-1-5923-3792-7   ISBN 978-1-5923-3791-0   ISBN 978-1-5923-3872-6   ISBN 978-1-5923-3871-9   ISBN 978-1-5923-3942-6